"This is not just another book about dieting, but rather a simple ten-step approach to improve the relationship between food and one's mind, body, and soul! The book promotes the principles that will maximize psychological and physical health to improve quantity and quality of life—something that I have promoted and written about for the past thirty-five years. This work should prove to be extremely helpful to many patients, including my own, and to the general public. I highly recommend it!"

—**Carl "Chip" Lavie, MD, FACC, FESPM**, medical director of cardiac rehabilitation and prevention, and director of exercise laboratories at John Ochsner Heart and Vascular Institute, and professor of medicine at Ochsner Clinical School, UQ School of Medicine

"*The Intuitive Eating Workbook*, written by *Health at Every Size* advocates Evelyn Tribole and Elyse Resch is an invaluable tool on your journey to developing a peaceful and satisfying relationship with food, mind, and body. It explains the principles of intuitive eating in a clear and inviting way, and offers a wealth of thought-provoking and effective exercises that help readers tune into their bodies' signals, and challenge distorted thoughts about food and body. This book will be a treasured resource for the general public and for health professionals as well."

—**Linda Bacon, PhD**, author of *Body Respect* and *Health at Every Size*

"*The Intuitive Eating Workbook* takes the wisdom of intuitive eating to a practical, informative self-help format. It is a perfect stand-alone workbook, as well as a supportive tool for work with patients. With activities that build resilience from a steady base of self-care, positive embodiment, and understanding, this book makes a deeper connection with your body and a healthier relationship with food completely accessible."

—**Catherine Cook-Cottone, PhD**, associate professor, licensed psychologist, and author of *Mindfulness and Yoga for Self-Regulation*

"With *The Intuitive Eating Workbook*, Tribole and Resch have created an empowering resource, not only for those who wish to embrace and practice intuitive eating, but also for health care professionals seeking to provide support. *The Intuitive Eating Workbook* provides a concise review of the foundational principles with references to supporting research and thoughtful exercises designed to promote attunement, self-care, and body appreciation. Tribole and Resch infuse each page with compassion and the unique perspective of their combined professional experience, making this a welcome healing tool for laypersons and professionals alike."

—**Paige O'Mahoney, MD, CHWC**, coauthor of *Helping Patients Outsmart Overeating*, certified Intuitive Eating counselor, and founder of Deliberate Life Wellness, LLC

"Evelyn and Elyse have done it again! I highly recommend *The Intuitive Eating Workbook*. Full freedom from food and body image problems is absolutely possible."

—**Jenni Schaefer**, author of *Goodbye Ed, Hello Me*; *Life Without Ed*; and coauthor of *Almost Anorexic*

"From the dangers of dieting and weight cycling to learning body respect and total self-care, this workbook covers all the bases of intuitive eating for both novices and those who need a bit more help along the way. Although dieticians generally teach us the 'what' of eating, Tribole and Resch write about the 'why' and 'how' of it as well as any seasoned eating disorders therapists."

—**Karen R. Koenig, MEd, LCSW**, author of *The Food and Feelings Workbook* and six other books on eating

"Evelyn Tribole and Elyse Resch's *The Intuitive Eating Workbook* is a must-have for anyone who wants to improve their relationship with food! Its practical, easy-to-read format walks you step-by-step through the process of learning to use your internal wisdom to enjoy eating food in a peaceful, healthy way. A fantastic resource for health care professionals."

—**Susan Albers**, psychologist and *New York Times* bestselling author of *EatQ*, *Eating Mindfully*, and *50 Ways to Soothe Yourself Without Food*

"Intuitive eating is both revolutionary and utterly logical. This is an invaluable guide to anyone who has ever struggled with food. In fact, I believe *anyone* would benefit from utilizing this resource as it directly challenges both our individual food issues, and those endemic to our culture. This is the end of dieting, for everyone."

—**Kelsey Miller**, author of *Big Girl*

"*The Intuitive Eating Workbook* is the perfect must-read, must-experience, and must-use supplement to Evelyn and Elyse's game-changing book, *Intuitive Eating*. The workbook models a dialect of compassion that makes each exercise accessible and—pun intended—digestible for all. *The Intuitive Eating Workbook* is *The Artist's Way* of health, offering keys to long-term, sustainable self-care, recognizing that eating is bigger than simply food itself. As Evelyn and Elyse say in the workbook, 'You are the expert of your own body,' an obvious and still radical notion that can both enhance our own lives, and also change the world at large."

—**Caroline Rothstein, MS**, writer, performer, activist, and educator

"Recovery from stress eating and body shame isn't about becoming a new person; it's a process that takes you back to the healthy, safe place you once knew as a child, before dreams of happiness through weight loss made you lose your way. *The Intuitive Eating Workbook* breaks down a potentially scary journey into practical, even enjoyable, steps. It's like you're on the yellow brick road, and Tribole and Resch are your ever-supportive sidekicks, warning you of pitfalls and boosting you when you struggle. Add in a catchy tune, and find your way back to where you always belonged."

—**Jessica Setnick, MS, RD, CEDRD**, author of *The Eating Disorders Clinical Pocket Guide* and *Eating Disorders Boot Camp*, and cofounder of the International Federation of Eating Disorder Dietitians

The

INTUITIVE
EATING
Workbook

Principles for Nourishing a
Healthy Relationship with Food

EVELYN TRIBOLE, MS, RDN
ELYSE RESCH, MS, RDN

New Harbinger Publications, Inc.

Publisher's Note

Distributed in Canada by Raincoast Books

Copyright © 2017 by Evelyn Tribole and Elyse Resch
        New Harbinger Publications, Inc.
        5674 Shattuck Avenue
        Oakland, CA 94609
        www.newharbinger.com

Intuitive Eating Assessment Scale–2 is adapted from Tylka, T. L., & Kroon Van Diest, A. M. (2013). The Intuitive Eating Scale–2: Item refinement and psychometric evaluation with college women and men. *Journal of Counseling Psychology*, 60(1), 137-153. http://dx.doi.org/10.1037/a0030893. Copyright © 2013 American Psychological Association. Adapted with permission.

Cover design by Amy Shoup

Acquired by Ryan Buresh

Edited by Jennifer Eastman

Library of Congress Cataloging-in-Publication Data on file

20   19   18

10   9   8   7   6

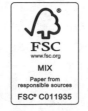
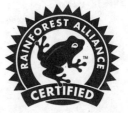

We dedicate this workbook to our past and present clients and future Intuitive Eaters. May you have dignity, health, and happiness—regardless of your shape or size— and may you never doubt your inner wisdom.

Contents

Acknowledgments

We are grateful to many people, including—but not limited to—the following:

David Hale Smith, Inkwell Management, LLC, our agent, for championing our work and his associate, Liz Parker, for her swift attention to detail.

Ryan Buresh, our acquisitions editor, for his enthusiastic vision; Jennifer Eastman, our copy editor, for her patience and diligent help; and the New Harbinger Publications editorial team for their guidance. Susan Albers, PsyD, for endorsing us and introducing us to New Harbinger Publications. St. Martin's Press, for graciously allowing us to reprint parts of *Intuitive Eating*.

Tracy Tylka, PhD, for putting Intuitive Eating on the research map and validating its many components.

The following researchers for sharing their tools and in sight:

Kristin Neff, PhD; Linda Bacon, PhD; Deb Bugard, PhD; Carl Lavie, MD; Catherine Cook-Cottone, PhD; Janet Polivy, PhD; C. Peter Herman, PhD; Ellen Satter, MS, RDN, MSSW; Susie Ohrbach; Jane Hirschmann, PhD and Carol Munter; Lauren Mellin, PhD; Rachel Calgero, PhD; Diane Neumark-Sztainer, PhD, MPH, RD; Traci Mann, PhD; Leann Birch, PhD.

To the following communities and individuals for advocating Intuitive Eating:

Health at Every Size, Certified Intuitive Eating Counselors, and the Intuitive Eating On-line Community.

Arlene Drake, PhD, LMFT, for her constant and nurturing support and advice throughout this project. (ER)

Pablo Nardi, for his unwavering support and basic goodness. (ET)

Shazi Shabatian, MS, RDN (Associate), and the members of the professional group I supervise, for their input and encouragement. (ER)

Samantha Mullen for her reliable and constant help with all Intuitive Eating projects. (ET)

Foreword

Congratulations on picking up this workbook. You may be sick of dieting, with all of its rules and stipulations. You may feel overwhelmed by dieting's promises, which give no lasting return. You may be tired of being preoccupied with food, as it consumes your valuable time and zaps your energy. You may be frustrated with hating your body, always feeling that you are fighting against it. You may desire an alternative way of relating to food, eating, and your body, one that is characterized by kindness rather than criticism. You want help. Or perhaps you know someone struggling with these issues, and you want to help him or her.

With the *Intuitive Eating Workbook*, by Evelyn Tribole and Elyse Resch, you will be working toward freedom from these issues. You will learn about how to cultivate a healthy relationship with food and your body. This will give you satisfying eating experiences, self-compassion, enhanced well-being, and respect for your body and mind.

Tribole and Resch are the ideal people to take you on this journey. They created Intuitive Eating, defined as a flexible style of eating in which you largely follow your internal sensations of hunger and satiety to gauge when to eat, what to eat, and when to stop eating. Following Intuitive Eating builds trust in your body. To be clear, Intuitive Eating is a process of *relearning* instincts we once knew. We are born Intuitive Eaters, but cultural messages to diet and lose weight often infiltrate our minds and sway us away from listening to our bodies. Thus, Intuitive Eating stands in contrast to dieting, which entails rigidly using external rules to determine when, what, and how much to eat. Following dieting plans erodes trust in your body.

Tribole and Resch successfully created the ten principles of Intuitive Eating to facilitate the healing of their clients' problematic relationships with food and their bodies. The authors published their first book on Intuitive Eating in 1995, and later editions, which included updated information and new chapters, appeared in 2003 and 2012. There is also an audiobook, released in 2009, which is not a verbatim reading of the book, but a discussion format with guided practices for all of the Intuitive Eating principles. I read their first volume in 2001, when I was a graduate student in counseling psychology and intern at a college counseling center. I used the ten principles to help my clients adopt a more adaptive relationship with food and their bodies. Once I witnessed Intuitive Eating's benefits in clinical settings, I wanted to conduct research on it to answer an important question. Is Intuitive Eating adaptive for us all?

To find an answer, I created a scale to assess Intuitive Eating and validated it with college and community samples of women and men. From this research, we have learned that Intuitive Eating is associated with a whole host of benefits, including enhanced satisfaction with life, self-compassion, self-esteem, optimism, and body appreciation. Intuitive eating also is associated with lower markers of distress, such as disordered eating, food preoccupation, food-related anxiety, body dissatisfaction, binge eating, uncontrolled eating, and depression. Although weight loss is not the goal of Intuitive Eating, research has found that it is also related to a lower body fat percentage and a lower body mass index. To date, over sixty articles tout its advantages. There you have it—there is a large and growing research base that supports Intuitive Eating as beneficial for your mind, body, and soul.

Within this workbook, Tribole and Resch explain the fundamentals of why Intuitive Eating will move you toward enhanced well-being, while dieting will move you in the opposite direction. When doing so, they integrate up-to-date research that justifies the inclusion of each principle. Yet Tribole and Resch don't stop there. They lead you through a series of thoughtful activities and reflections that cultivate each of the ten principles of Intuitive Eating. Underlying these principles is the nurturing of *attunement*—the ability to be in touch with what is going on in your body—and honoring your body through engaging in self-care and self-compassion. As Tribole and Resch emphasize, these principles are meant to be practiced regularly, and the activities in this workbook provide innovative and practical ways to achieve this goal. The authors also help you identify factors that disrupt attunement and self-care, thereby usurping Intuitive Eating, and they help you to generate strategies to move past these disruptions. Thus, this workbook serves as a valuable tool for how to implement the ten principles of Intuitive Eating within your daily life.

—Tracy L. Tylka, PhD, FAED
　　Department of Psychology
　　The Ohio State University
　　Fellow, Academy for Eating Disorders
　　Associate Editor, *Body Image: An International Journal of Research*

Introduction

The well-intentioned pursuit of wellness and a so-called healthy weight has been hijacked by a confluence of factors, and healthy eating has evolved into a near religious endeavor, with morality and absolution attained through consuming the "proper diet." Public health policy has contributed to this dilemma by declaring a war on obesity; a holy war, if you will, which has led to both weight stigma and a flourishing dieting industry—to the tune of nearly $60 billion per year.

Fearmongering, in the name of health, in front of the backdrop of an appearance-based culture, has triggered the perception that we are one bite away from a disaster. It's a cultural neurosis; the fork has become akin to a loaded gun—just one wrong move pulls the trigger. This creates a perpetual background anxiety at the kitchen table and every time you eat: *Eater beware—you are only a bite away from a heart attack or obesity.*

It's no wonder that people are driven to popular eating crazes, such as "clean eating" and fad dieting, all in the name of health. But this pursuit is creating more problems. A substantial body of research shows that dieting is not sustainable and leads to a host of problems, including eating disorders, food and body preoccupation, distraction from other personal health goals, reduced self-esteem, weight stigmatization, discrimination, and—paradoxically—weight *gain.*

As a result, people are weary of dieting and yet terrified of eating. People don't know how to eat anymore. They are ashamed of their bodies and don't trust that their bodies "work." The pleasure of eating has been stolen. Intuitive Eating—a concept we created in 1995, based on evaluating hundreds of studies, in addition to our clinical experience—is the solution to this growing dilemma.

What Is Intuitive Eating?

Intuitive Eating is a dynamic mind-body integration of instinct, emotion, and rational thought. It is a personal process of honoring your health by paying attention to the messages of your body and meeting your physical and emotional needs. It is an inner journey of discovery that puts you front and center; *you* are the expert of your own body. After all, only *you* know your thoughts, feelings, and experiences. Only you know how hungry you are and what food or meal will satisfy you. No diet plan or guru could possibly know these things.

There are ten principles of Intuitive Eating, which work in two key ways. Some of them help you gain body attunement—that is, the ability to hear (and thus respond to) the physical sensations that arise within your body, such as biological cues of hunger and fullness—and other principles work by removing the obstacles to body attunement.

Cultivating Attunement. The ability to perceive bodily sensations is known as *interoceptive awareness*, which is critical for attunement. This is because biological states, such as having a full bladder or feeling sleepy or hungry, have a physical sensation. Even emotional states have a physical sensation, which can be very subtle. Being attuned to the physical sensations of your body gives you powerful information into your physiological and psychological state, which helps you determine what you should do to meet your needs. Perhaps you need to sleep; maybe you need to eat or play, or maybe you just need a break. Your body knows! It's rather profound—that all of this information is available to you just by listening and paying attention to your body.

Removing Obstacles to Attunement. If, rather than listening to your body, you have instead repeatedly followed popular diet crazes, you may find yourself thinking that you don't know how to eat anymore. You may be feeling confused, conflicted, and mistrustful of your body. That's why the principles of Intuitive Eating also work to remove the obstacles to body attunement. Obstacles to interoceptive awareness usually originate from your mind, in the form of thoughts, beliefs, and rules—such as rules about what you *should* or *should not* eat, beliefs about what a healthy body *should* look like, and judgmental thoughts about *good* food versus *bad* food. Part of the antidote is challenging these beliefs, rules, and thoughts, while cultivating a kind and compassionate view along your journey to becoming an Intuitive Eater.

Cultivating a self-compassionate viewpoint is vitally important on this journey. It's about looking at your situation with kindness, because having compassion for yourself creates an inviting atmosphere for learning and moving forward.

If there were an eleventh principle of Intuitive Eating, it would be self-care. If you are not getting your basic needs met (such as enough sleep), it can interfere with body attunement. At best, it may make it difficult to hear, let alone respond to, the messages of your body in a timely manner. At worst, you might find yourself turning to food to self-soothe and cope. That's why you will be learning a lot about self-care throughout this workbook.

Benefits of Intuitive Eating

When we wrote our first book, *Intuitive Eating,* over twenty years ago, we had no idea that our concept would generate many studies. To date, there have been over sixty studies on Intuitive Eating from around the world, which show many associated health benefits, including increased well-being, lower risk of eating disorders, and improved biomarkers, such as blood sugar and cholesterol. Intuitive Eaters also enjoy eating a variety of foods and have better interoceptive awareness and psychological hardiness.

One of the seminal studies was by psychologist and researcher Tracy Tylka from Ohio State University, who created the Intuitive Eating Assessment Scale [IEAS] and validated it though a study involving over four thousand men and women (Tylka 2006; Tylka and Kroon Van Diest 2013). Near the end of this introduction, you will have an opportunity to see where you fall on this assessment tool.

Because of its many health benefits, Intuitive Eating has been embraced by state public health departments, employee wellness programs, college student health programs, and many other programs that promote health and well-being. At many universities, *Intuitive Eating* is a required text in courses in a number of academic departments, including nutrition, psychology, and health education. Finally, eating disorder treatment programs are incorporating the principles as a significant part of their treatment protocol.

The benefits of Intuitive Eating have been popularized beyond the research world, with mounting interest from the media, health professionals, corporate wellness programs, and the readers of our books. Consequently, we have been inundated with requests for a workbook on the Intuitive Eating principles. Interest in this workbook has come from both consumers, who want to hone their Intuitive Eating skills, and health professionals and researchers, who are seeking practical exercises for their clients.

Who Will Benefit from the Intuitive Eating Workbook? This workbook can be completed individually, with a counselor, or within a group setting. Special note to those with medical conditions and eating disorders—we strongly recommend that you complete this workbook in conjunction with your health treatment team.

What Should You Expect? Practicing the activities through this book will help you achieve a healthy relationship with food, mind, and your body. We call this achievement *authentic health*. We say that it is *authentic* because it reflects your inner state of attunement with your body and mind, and—equally—it is integrated with health guidelines from scientific consensus (see figure I.1).

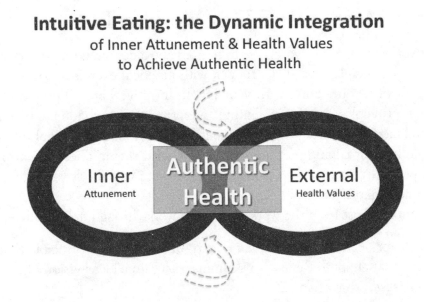

Figure I.1.   Intuitive Eating: the dynamic integration.
Adapted with permission from Catherine Cook-Cottone, SUNY Buffalo.
Reprinted with permission from Tribole and Resch 2012 / St. Martin's Press.

It's important to keep in mind that health includes a wide variety of factors. "Health is a state of complete physical, mental, and social well-being, and not merely the absence of disease or infirmity. The enjoyment of the highest attainable standard of health is one of the fundamental rights of every human being without distinction of race, religion, political belief, economic or social condition" (World Health Organization 2006).

When we talk to people about Intuitive Eating, they often ask, "Will I lose weight?" By following the ten principles of Intuitive Eating, you will normalize your relationship with eating and your body. Weight loss may or may not be a side effect. If you focus on weight loss, that preoccupation will interfere with your ability to make choices based on your intuitive signals, and it will place focus on appearance rather than inner wisdom. There is also a profound body of research—based on millions of people, cumulatively—that shows that weight, especially the body mass index, is not a good indicator of health (Lavie 2014; Ross et al. 2015; Friedemann Smith, Heneghan, and Ward 2015; Tomiyama et al. 2016). Furthermore, a scientific review has concluded that the pursuit of weight loss alone is linked to diminished health (Tylka et al. 2014). On the other hand, placing the focus on healthy lifestyle behaviors, rather than on weight, provides health benefits with or without weight loss (Ross et al. 2015; Bacon and Aphramor 2011). It is time that public health policy focuses on health and healthy behaviors. Period. Weight is not a health behavior. Intuitive Eating is about cultivating a healthy relationship with food, mind, and body—it's about self-care and body appreciation, regardless of size—not about the pursuit of weight loss.

Getting the Most Out of This Workbook

We hope that you will find this workbook to not only be a comprehensive review of Intuitive Eating and its ten principles but also a rudder, with practical exercises, to steer you through the winding path of reconnecting with your innate Intuitive Eater. This workbook is organized by the ten principles of Intuitive Eating, one principle per chapter. There are exercises to challenge and modify distorted thoughts about food and your body and also to identify your emotions, while finding coping mechanisms to deal with them. There are also attunement exercises and practices, to help you to hear the messages your body is sending you and to respond in a timely manner.

You will gain the most from the workbook if you work through it carefully:

- Each chapter begins with a one-paragraph summary of the principle that will be discussed in that chapter. Review this summary to gain a clear vision of the intention of the exercises in that chapter.

- Commit to writing out or performing each activity. Sometimes you may need to do an exercise more than once—as a practice. It's no different than when you learn to swim or play a musical instrument; sometimes you need repetition and practice to really get it, even though you understand the mechanics. You need experience working with your mind and body in order to cultivate trust in the inner wisdom from your body.

- As a useful adjunct, read the most recent edition of *Intuitive Eating*. While this workbook can stand alone, we think that you will find it helpful to read more of the rationale behind each principle, as well as detailed discussion of the case studies and research.

One of the great benefits of this workbook is that it gives readers a solid and detailed framework for practicing Intuitive Eating. An intellectual understanding of the concepts and principles of Intuitive Eating is important, but it is not the same as having the experience of eating intuitively. Attuning and responding to the needs of your body takes practice and patience—it does not come from merely reading about it.

We invite you to partake in two introductory activities. First, there is the Handwriting Metaphor Activity, which will help you understand the importance of the three *p*'s of learning to become an Intuitive Eater: *paying attention*, *patience*, and *practice*. Then you will complete a brief Intuitive Eating Assessment Scale.

Handwriting Metaphor Activity

There are three parts to this activity. You will need a pen or pencil for this exercise. It's important to take your time for this exercise and, preferably, complete it in a quiet environment, free from distraction.

Part 1. Write Your Name

Place the pen or pencil in your dominant hand (right hand, for most people). Then write your name below, and take as much time as you need. *Pay attention* to how the pen feels in your hand as you write.

_____

Next, switch hands. Put your pen or pencil in your nondominant hand (left hand, for most people) and write your name below. Remember to take your time and *pay attention* to how the pen feels in this hand.

_____

Part 2. Compare and Contrast the Signatures

1. Look at your two signatures. Is there a quality difference between the signatures written with the dominant versus the nondominant hand? How so?

    _____

    _____

    _____

2. Did it feel awkward *holding* the pen in the nondominant hand? How did it *feel physically* when you were *writing* with your nondominant hand? Compare and contrast the physical sensation of holding the pen in your dominant versus nondominant hand?

    _____

    _____

    _____

3. What were your thoughts as you were writing? Perhaps you had thoughts of frustration and judgment: *My writing looks like that of a first-grader.*

    _____

    _____

    _____

4. What were your emotional feelings? Perhaps you were feeling impatient, judgmental, intrigued, embarrassed, fearful, or amused?

_____

_____

_____

5. Did you have the belief or expectation that your writing should appear of the same quality, even if your nondominant hand has had less experience?

_____

_____

_____

Part 3. Discussion and Processing

Both of your hands have access to the same brain, which possesses the knowledge of how to write and spell your name. Yet, for the majority of people, there is a marked difference in the quality of the writing, which reflects the significance of experience or practice.

Learning how to become an Intuitive Eater is a lot like learning how to write with your nondominant hand—it takes practice. Intellectual knowledge is not enough. If you have not had much experience listening and responding to your body cues in a timely manner, it will take patience and practice. If you have spent years dieting and creating food rules, it will take time to challenge and deconstruct those rules and beliefs, which can interfere with Intuitive Eating.

Reflect upon your eating experiences. Do you have much experience in *paying attention* to and honoring your body? What might that mean for you in terms of cultivating *patience* and compassion with the process?

_____

_____

_____

_____

Like the Handwriting Metaphor Activity, the exercises in this workbook will help you connect with your body sensations, thoughts, feelings, and beliefs and help you to *pay attention* to them as well as *practicing* new ways to work with them. Doing these exercises will help you find ways to honor yourself, figure out what you really need in life, and provide you with long-lasting experiences, which will lead to a deep trust in your body, your mind, and your soul. Please remember to be kind and *patient* with yourself on your journey to becoming an Intuitive Eater.

Intuitive Eating Assessment Scale—2

This assessment is adapted with permission from Tracy Tylka's research on Tribole and Resch's model of Intuitive Eating (Tylka 2006; Tylka and Kroon Van Diest 2013; Tribole and Resch 1995, 2012).

In the following table, statements are grouped into the three core characteristics of Intuitive Eaters. Answer yes or no for each statement. If you are unsure of how to respond to a statement at first, that's okay—you might be somewhere between a clear yes or no. But most people will lean in one direction or the other. Read the statement a few times and consider if the description *usually* applies to you. Is it mostly yes or no?

Yes	No	Section 1. Unconditional Permission to Eat
		1. I try to avoid certain foods high in fat, carbs, or calories.
		2. If I am craving a certain food, I don't allow myself to have it.
		3. I get mad at myself for eating something unhealthy.
		4. I have forbidden foods that I don't allow myself to eat.
		5. I don't allow myself to eat what food I desire at the moment.
		6. I follow eating rules or diet plans that dictate what, when, and how to eat.

		Section 2. Eating for Physical Rather Than Emotional Reasons
		1. I find myself eating when I'm feeling emotional (i.e., anxious, sad, depressed), even when I'm not physically hungry.
		2. I find myself eating when I am lonely, even when I'm not physically hungry.
		3. I use food to help me soothe my negative emotions.
		4. I find myself eating when I am stressed out, even when I'm not physically hungry.
		5. I am not able to cope with my negative emotions (e.g., anxiety and sadness) without turning to food for comfort.
		6. When I am bored, I eat just for something to do.
		7. When I am lonely, I turn to food for comfort.
		8. I have difficulty finding ways to cope with stress and anxiety, other than by eating.
		Section 3. Reliance on Internal Hunger and Satiety Cues
		1. I trust my body to tell me *when* to eat.
		2. I trust my body to tell me *what* to eat.
		3. I trust my body to tell me *how much* to eat.
		4. I rely on my hunger signals to tell me when to eat.
		5. I rely on my fullness (satiety) signals to tell me when to stop eating.
		6. I trust my body to tell me when to stop eating.
		Section 4. Body-Food Choice Congruence
		1. Most of the time, I desire to eat nutritious foods.
		2. I mostly eat foods that make my body perform efficiently (well).
		3. I mostly eat foods that give my body energy and stamina.

Scoring

For Sections 1 and 2. Add up your yes responses and write it in the left-hand column of the table below. Each yes statement indicates an area that likely needs some work.

Total Yes Responses	Section
	Section 1. Unconditional Permission to Eat (six statements)
	Section 2. Eating for Physical Rather than Emotional Reasons (eight statements)

For Sections 3 and 4. Add up your no responses and write it in the left-hand column of the table below. Each no statement indicates an area that likely needs some work.

Total No Responses	Section
	Section 3. Reliance on Internal Hunger and Satiety Cues (six statements)
	Section 4. Body-Food Choice Congruence (four statements)

It will be helpful to periodically retake this assessment to help gauge your progress. You can record and compare your scores below.

Section	Date	Date	Date	Date
	Score Totals			
1. Unconditional Permission to Eat				
2. Eating for Physical Rather than Emotional Reasons				
3. Reliance on Internal Hunger and Satiety Cues				
4. Body-Food Choice Congruence				

Please do not fret if you answered yes to many of the statements in the first two sections or have a lot of responses of no in the last two sections. This is simply an assessment to see where you are at now—not a judgment! Consider that your responses merely indicate how much this workbook will help you. Imagine how you will feel when you are genuinely able to change your responses—the freedom from food and body anxiety, with self-confidence and inner trust of your body's innate wisdom.

In the first chapter, you will learn how to reject the dieting mentality, which is a critical first step toward inner peace and freedom in becoming an Intuitive Eater.

CHAPTER 1

Principle One
Reject the Diet Mentality

Throw out the diet books and magazine articles that offer you false hope of losing weight quickly, easily, and permanently. Get angry at the lies that have led you to feel as if you were a failure every time a new diet stopped working and you gained back all of the weight. If you allow even one small hope to linger that a new and better diet might be lurking around the corner, it will prevent you from being free to rediscover Intuitive Eating.

If dieting programs had to stand up to the same scrutiny as medications, they would never be allowed for public consumption. Imagine, for example, taking a cholesterol medication that improved your blood results for a few weeks but, in the long run, caused your arteries to clog. Would you really embark on a dieting program (even a so-called sensible diet) if you knew that it could cause you to gain more weight and affect your emotional well-being?

Dieting Leads to Weight Gain

Many people are aware that dieting doesn't work in the long run, but most are surprised to learn that dieting actually increases your risk for gaining even *more* weight. Since the late 1940s, a large body of research has shown that the act of dieting promotes weight gain in a variety of age groups, from children and teens to adults.

There are profound biological mechanisms at play that trigger rebound weight gain from dieting. As far as your cells are concerned, they are being subjected to a famine, and they'll do anything to survive. Your cells have no idea that you are choosing to restrict your calories (or some group of foods) for weight loss. One well-known survival adaptation they have is to slow down metabolism. A six-year follow-up study of contestants on the weight-loss show *The Biggest Loser* showed that, compared to their baseline, the contestants' metabolisms were suppressed by an average of five hundred calories (Fothergill et al. 2016). Predictably, they gained back a significant amount of their weight.

Another way the body survives dieting is by cannibalizing its own muscle. That's because energy is so important that the body will destroy its own muscle to burn as fuel (the muscle is converted to carbohydrates). That's like being so poor that you can't afford the heating bill or to buy wood for a fire, so you burn your kitchen cabinets for warmth. The *Biggest Loser* study also showed this effect. The contestants actually had more lean tissue at the beginning of the competition (Fothergill et al. 2016)! Six years later, their muscle was not restored to their baseline levels. They also had lower levels of leptin—a hormone that triggers feelings of fullness.

Fat overshooting is another way the body tries to survive the dieting process (Dulloo, Jacquet, and Montani 2012). In essence, the loss of both fat and lean muscle tissue triggers the body to gain more weight in the form of body fat to survive. Hormonal changes also make you more hungry and preoccupied with food.

Altogether, these powerful compensatory adaptations make sustained weight loss extremely difficult for most people. This makes for a great business model (built-in repeat business) for the nearly $60 billion-per-year weight-loss industry. It's the only business that produces a product that doesn't work but is not blamed for this failure—the consumers blame themselves.

The Paradox of So-Called Healthy Weight

We have long-argued that there is little support for the position that weight loss is mandatory in order to achieve health benefits from lifestyle changes.

—Ross et al. 2015

Perhaps you have pursued weight loss for health reasons and believe you have no choice but to diet. Maybe your doctor told you to lose weight in order to be healthy. There is a body of research that shows otherwise.

In his book *The Obesity Paradox*, cardiologist and researcher Carl J. Lavie describes how the war on obesity has actually created bigger health problems. High-quality studies on millions of people show that being at a lower weight does not confer better health or outcomes. He concludes: "Health should not be measured by a number on the scale or the size of your jeans" (Lavie 2014, 230). Two recent studies also came to a similar conclusion:

- A UCLA study found that fifty-four million Americans are labeled obese or overweight, according to their BMI, but they are actually healthy (Tomiyama et al. 2016).

- Overweight patients with type 2 diabetes were placed on weight-loss diets and supervised over six years by physicians; a control group of similar patients received no treatment. The researchers were stunned to discover that the dieters had a worse prognosis than the control group, who had maintained their *overweight* status (Køster-Rasmussen et al. 2016).

The pursuit of weight loss, even in the name of health, perpetuates body-weight bias and stigma. These are forms of prejudice that make assumptions about your health and value based solely on your size. Sadly, weight discrimination, like discrimination based on race, has a negative impact on health (Bacon and Aphramor 2011).

Healthy behaviors are important regardless of size. That's why there is a growing movement called Health at Every Size (HAES), which shifts the focus from weight management to healthy behaviors that are sustainable (Bacon and Aphramor 2011; Tylka et al. 2014). This approach challenges the notion that your BMI reflects your health practices, health status, or moral character (Tylka et al. 2014).

Dieting Hurts Your Psychological Health and Well-Being

Many of our clients romanticize their first diet like a first love—it was so easy and effortless. The weight just came off. But that first dieting experience is the seduction trap that launches the cycle of weight loss and gain. With each diet, your body adapts and learns how to survive, making it even more difficult to lose weight. With each failed weight-loss attempt, a learned helplessness becomes stronger, resulting in poor self-efficacy and empowerment (Ross et al. 2015; Tylka et al. 2014). Consequently, many of our patients feel like failures—but it is the system of dieting that has failed them.

It's no wonder that dieting also increases the risk of eating disorders, including binge eating. Dieting contributes to body dissatisfaction, food and body preoccupation, food cravings, distraction from other personal health goals, reduced self-esteem, and weight stigmatization and discrimination (Bacon and Aphramor 2011; Tomiyama et al. 2016; Tylka et al. 2014; Mann 2015).

When the dieting mentality is engaged, your eating decisions are dictated by the diet rules, which mandate what you eat, regardless of your food preferences, energy needs, hunger, and so forth, all of which can trigger feelings of deprivation. No diet plan could possibily know your hunger level or the foods that satisfy you. The dieting rules also trigger an inner rebellion, because they are an assault on your personal autonomy and boundaries.

Even when you are not on a diet, your mind may still have the insidious mentality of dieting—the *shoulds* and *should nots* of eating. This mental construct creates an obstacle to Intuitive Eating.

Intuitive Eating is based on attunement and uses the direct experience of your body. Is your body experiencing hunger? Is your body comfortably full and satisfied? It's a process of listening and responding to the needs of your body. The dieting mentality erodes trust in your body, because "the rules" micromanage and dictate your food choices, *regardless of how you feel*. This creates a cognitive dissonance, a clash between what you are experiencing to be true and what you're told to do, which leads to confusion about eating, with the common lament: "I don't know how to eat any more."

The activities in this chapter will help you to

- cultivate self-compassion;

- explore your dieting history;

- recognize and acknowledge how dieting has interfered with your life, both physically and psychologically;

- explore the benefits of letting go of dieting;

- identify the diet mentality's traits and thinking; and

- get rid of the tools of dieting.

Cultivating Self-Compassion

It's important to keep in mind that every eating experience you have, whether perceived as negative or positive, is an opportunity to learn about your body. Intuitive Eating is not a pass or fail process—it's a learning experience. A toddler learning to walk will dawdle, stumble, and fall, but parents delight in each and every step and respond with compassionate encouragement. We can't imagine a parent scolding a little tyke who takes a misstep and falls: "You idiot, get up!" Similarly, it's important for you to cultivate self-compassion rather than shame and blame. Research indicates that adopting a self-compassionate stance toward difficult experiences related to your body may help facilitate Intuitive Eating and overcome body dissatisfaction (Schoenefeld and Webb 2013; Albertson, Neff, and Dill-Shackleford 2015).

Self-compassion is associated with well-being, increased feelings of happiness, and greater personal initiative to make needed changes in your life (Neff 2003, 2016; Neff and Costigan 2014). Some people have expressed concern that self-compassion might be used as an excuse for overindulgence or letting yourself off the hook, but this is not the case. Self-compassion is simply having a neutral but understanding consideration of yourself and your actions. Research has shown that self-compassion helps people overcome their guilt with their eating choices (Adams and Leary 2007). Self-compassion can thus help promote change. This is because self-compassionate individuals do not criticize or bully themselves when they make mistakes. This makes it easier for them to admit vulnerability and mistakes, change unproductive behaviors, and take on new challenges, such as Intuitive Eating.

So before we begin exploring your dieting history and related issues, let's begin the work of cultivating compassion. The following exercises are based on the research and exercises of Kristin Neff (http://self-compassion.org), and adapted with her permission.

Self-Compassion Exercises

1. Think about times when you were struggling with your eating. How do you typically respond? Write down what you typically do and what you say to yourself. Be sure to notice the tone of your thoughts—are they harsh and intense or gentle and kind?

   _____

   _____

   _____

   _____

2. If you had a dear friend or loved one who was struggling with his or her eating, how would you respond? Write down what you would say to your friend. Also note the tone you would use with a friend or loved one—is it harsh or kind?

   _____

   _____

   _____

   _____

3. Is there a difference between the way you would talk to your friend and the way you talk to yourself? If yes, what factors or fears come into play that lead you to treat yourself and others so differently?

   _____

   _____

   _____

   _____

4. How might things change if you responded kindly to yourself (like the way you typically respond to a close friend who is struggling)?

   _____

   _____

   _____

   _____

5. Bullying and fearmongering in the name of health do not work and may actually worsen your health in the long run. Do you use self-criticism or self-bullying as motivators for your eating issues? Reflect on a recent difficult situation with your eating or body. As you call the situation to mind, see if you can actually feel the emotional discomfort in your body. Describe how this feels.

_____

_____

_____

_____

6. What compassionate words or phrases could you use to replace the inner bully? Think of a kinder, more supportive inner dialogue. It may help to think of what a caring friend would say to you when you are suffering. How does that make you feel emotionally and physically?

_____

_____

_____

_____

Your Dieting History

Over the years we have had many clients report that a particular diet really worked. Yet upon closer reflection, that was not the case at all. Our clients had temporarily lost weight, but then they regained all the weight (and often added even more, compared to their baseline).

The purpose of this section is to help you see the truth of your dieting history. While this worksheet looks at your weight history—the focal point of dieting—we want to stress that Intuitive Eating is not about scales and numbers. Intuitive Eating is not a diet! Dieting promises weight loss, and we want you to examine the truth of these promises. Did you lose weight permanently, or was it only temporary weight loss? Or are you like the millions of people who not only regained the weight they lost but also gained *more* weight (as has been shown in study after study)?

Dieting History Worksheet

Using the worksheet below, list your age at the time of the particular diet, your reason for dieting, the type of diet, the duration of the diet, whether you lost weight, and was there a rebound weight gain? You may use the "other" column to add your own notes.

Age	Reason for starting the diet	Type of diet	How long did you stay on the diet?	Did you lose weight?	If you lost weight, how long did you keep the weight off?	Did you regain the weight?	Did you regain more weight than you lost?	Other

Using the information from the Dieting History Worksheet, answer the following questions.

1. Consider why you started dieting. Did you feel pressure to lose weight from family, friends, or a physician?

   _____

   _____

2. How did your first diet feel? Was it easy, even effortless? How so?

   _____

   _____

3. What was the longest period of time that you sustained a weight loss from dieting?

   _____

   _____

4. What trend do you see with your body weight, since your first diet?

   _____

   _____

5. Currently, do you find it more difficult to stay on a diet—both mentally and physically?

   _____

   _____

6. How often have you said that a diet worked because you had a temporary weight loss? When you review your dieting history, was the weight loss ever permanent or did the weight gradually come back?

   _____

   _____

How Has Dieting Interfered with Your Life?

There is a huge cost to the pursuit of dieting, beyond financial. Dieting can cause a lot of harm to your behavioral and mental health, as well as your social, relationship, and physical health. The following inventory helps you to examine how dieting has affected you.

Inventory of How Dieting Has Interfered with Your Life

This list includes consequences that result from dieting. Check all that apply to you. Each column has space at the bottom to add consequences not listed here.

Physical Symptoms	Social Symptoms	Psychological Symptoms	Behavioral Symptoms
☐ Weight gain.	☐ I eat differently when others are present.	☐ I worry about my eating.	☐ If I break a food rule, I eat even more of it.
☐ Blunted metabolism.	☐ I compare my food to what others are eating, in quantity and type of foods.	☐ I have strict rules about eating.	☐ If I eat too much, I make up for it by skipping a meal or eating less food at the next meal, even if I am hungry.
☐ Excessive cravings for carbs.		☐ I count calories, carbs, or other factors about food.	
☐ Blood sugar swings.	☐ I worry about what people think about my eating.	☐ I think of foods as "good" or "bad."	☐ I eat more food when I'm stressed.
☐ Disconnected from hunger cues.	☐ I worry about what people think about my body.	☐ I feel guilty if I eat a "bad" food.	☐ I exercise only to burn calories or lose weight.
☐ Disconnected from satiety cues.	☐ I try to eat the same type and quantity of food that others are eating.	☐ I have mood swings.	☐ I talk a lot about dieting, weight, and food.
☐ Chronically tired, even when sleeping well.		☐ I am afraid of feeling hungry.	☐ When I'm on vacation, I ignore my food rules and eat more than I need, no matter how full I feel.
☐ Hair loss (more than usual).	☐ I cancel social events because of the food or meals served.	☐ I am afraid of feeling too full.	
☐ If female: missed or inconsistent menses.	☐ I avoid eating in social situations.	☐ I don't trust my body.	☐ I engage in binge eating.
☐ Physical numbness.	☐ My behavior and beliefs about my eating and body have interfered with relationships.	☐ I am afraid that if I start eating "forbidden" foods, I won't stop eating.	☐ I avoid physical intimacy.
☐ Other:	☐ Other:	☐ I fantasize about food	☐ Other:
		☐ I am preoccupied by thoughts about what I eat and don't eat.	
		☐ Other:	

What Are the Personal Benefits of Letting Go of Dieting?

Answer the following questions, using information from both the Dieting History Worksheet and the inventory of how dieting has interfered with your life.

Part 1. The Different Costs of Dieting

1. How has dieting affected your social life?

   _____

   _____

   _____

   _____

2. How has dieting affected your eating behavior?

   _____

   _____

   _____

   _____

3. How has dieting affected your mind and mood?

   _____

   _____

   _____

   _____

4. What physical consequences have you experienced from dieting?

   _____

   _____

   _____

   _____

5. How much time and money have you spent in the pursuit of weight loss?

_____

_____

_____

_____

Part 2. Comparing Fantasy Thoughts with Your History

1. What kind of thoughts do you hold that may be fueling a fantasy of going on one last diet?

_____

_____

_____

_____

2. Considering your dieting history and the subsequent impact on your weight, eating behavior, social life, and mental state, what would be some reasons for you to let go of dieting, once and for all?

_____

_____

_____

_____

The Dangers of Weight Cycling

When you embark on diet after diet, it leads to weight fluctuations, which researchers call *weight cycling*. Weight cycling itself takes a toll on your physical and mental health. Research over the past twenty-five years has shown that weight cycling is inextricably linked to adverse physical health and psychological well-being (Dulloo, Jacquet, and Montani 2012; Tylka et al. 2014):

- The landmark Framingham Heart Study evaluated more than five thousand people over a thirty-two-year period and found that weight cycling was strongly linked to overall death rates, as well as mortality and morbidity related to heart disease.

- A weight-loss study from Korea found that women with a history of weight cycling lost more muscle but not more body fat, compared to women who did not experience weight cycling, despite having lost a similar amount of weight overall.

- The Nurses' Health Study 2 found that women with a history of weight cycling gained more weight over time and engaged in more binge eating than their counterparts.

- Weight cycling increases the risk of bone fractures from osteoporosis, gallstones, loss of muscle, high blood pressure, chronic inflammation, and some forms of cancer.

- Weight cycling has also been shown to be a predictor of subsequent weight gain in male athletes involved in weight-based sports such as boxing, wrestling, and weight lifting.

Letting Go of the Fantasy

Even when you are clear that dieting does not work for you and, moreover, that it causes harm, it can still be difficult to let go of the fantasy of weight loss and achieving a "new you":

1. What are your beliefs about weight loss, in general?

_____

_____

_____

_____

2. What are your beliefs about your own weight loss?

_____

_____

_____

_____

3. Where did these beliefs come from? What is their origin?

_____

_____

_____

_____

4. How do you fantasize life changing for you if you pursued weight loss?

_____

_____

_____

_____

5. How have your beliefs about weight loss affected you?

   A. Have you put some aspects of your life on hold until you lose weight (such as pursuing jobs, relationships, or activities)?

   _____

   _____

   _____

   _____

   B. Reflect upon your responses to question 5A. What would you need in order to explore your desired pursuits in your "here-and-now body"?

   _____

   _____

   _____

   _____

Holding on to the fantasy of weight loss can keep you stuck in the diet mentality, even when you do not plan to engage in dieting behavior.

Getting Rid of the Tools of Dieting

Weighing, measuring, and counting are external tools of dieting. And so is collecting dieting books and articles. Which of these tools or techniques might you still be using? Review the twenty statements below and place a check by those that apply to you.

	1. I count calories or points and try not to exceed a daily total of _____.
	2. I will not let myself eat a particular snack if it exceeds a certain number of calories or points.
	3. I will not let myself eat a particular meal if it exceeds a certain number of calories or points.
	4. When I eat out at restaurants, I choose entrees that have the lowest calories or points.
	5. I do not allow myself to drink beverages that have any calories.
	6. I choose physical activities and exercise based on the amount of calories it burns.
	7. I cannot eat a particular meal or food if I do not know the calories or points.
	8. I avoid eating foods that are high in carbohydrates such as bread, cereal, and pasta.
	9. I avoid eating foods that contain sugar.
	10. I avoid eating foods that contain fat.
	11. I weigh myself frequently.
	12. I measure my food to be sure I am not eating too many calories.
	13. I count the exact amount of food I need to eat (such as nuts or crackers), in order to be sure that I don't eat more than one serving or portion size.
	14. I weigh my food to be sure I am not eating too much.
	15. If I think I ate too much food, I will compensate by exercising more.
	16. I google articles on new diet plans and how to lose weight.
	17. I read blogs and websites about dieting and "thinspiration."
	18. I save books on various diets and dieting plans.
	19. I collect low-calorie recipes to help lose weight.
	20. I take supplements, including teas, which are supposed to burn fat, speed metabolism, or help lose weight.

Review the statements—the dieting tools—that you checked off. There may be a lot of them, and that's okay. It's important to start just where you are. We work with people all the time who use several tools to "keep their eating in check." With time, you will learn to let go of them, bringing you to a healthier relationship with eating. For now, select the three tools that you feel might be easiest to let go of.

1. Write down the first tool you choose to work on. Describe one step you could take to let go of it. (For example, when eating out, rather than selecting the lowest-calorie entrée, you could choose an entrée that would be satisfying to eat, regardless of calories.)

_____

_____

_____

_____

2. Write down the second tool and describe one step you could take to let go of it.

_____

_____

_____

_____

3. Write down the third tool and describe one step you could take to let go of it.

_____

_____

_____

_____

Dieting Mentality: Exploring the Hidden Forms of Dieting

Your self-critical dieting voice may be so familiar to you that you don't even notice it. This may make you inadvertently turn Intuitive Eating into another diet with rules and shoulds, which will leave you feeling stressed out and guilt-ridden. Because of this, it's important to learn to recognize the dieting mentality. You might not be following any official diet, but your mind might still be in the habit of using the language of dieting, which, in turn, can promote restrictive eating behaviors. Additionally, some eating plans are actually dieting plans, cleverly marketed under the guise of eating for your health. Review the statements below and place a check next to those that apply to you.

	1. I try not to eat any carbohydrates, especially grain-based foods such as cereal, rice, or pasta.
	2. I like to participate in juice cleanses.
	3. I usually describe a day of eating as either good or bad.
	4. If I eat dessert, I will need to exercise more.
	5. If I perceive that I ate too much at a particular meal, I will automatically eat less at the next meal, regardless of my hunger and fullness level.
	6. I view food as the enemy.
	7. I allow myself "cheat days," when I allow myself to eat whatever I want, regardless of my hunger and fullness level.
	8. I eat really carefully on weekdays and then eat whatever I like over the weekends, regardless of my hunger and fullness level.
	9. Once I eat a forbidden food, I think, *I blew it*, and then I eat whatever I want in larger quantities, regardless of my hunger and fullness level.
	10. If I am planning to go out for dinner, I cut back how much I eat during the day, regardless of my hunger and fullness level.
	11. I often choose the smallest portion of food for a meal or snack, regardless of my hunger and fullness level.
	12. If I don't exercise one day, I compensate by cutting back on what I eat, regardless of my hunger and fullness level.
	13. I feel guilty if I don't exercise, because it means that I did not burn off any calories.
	14. I participate in worksite weight-loss competitions and in food-restriction events, such as thirty-day challenges to cut out gluten or white flour or processed foods.
	15. I watch television shows like *The Biggest Loser* in order to inspire myself to lose weight.
	16. I like to talk about the calorie counts of foods.
	17. If I am at a luncheon or restaurant, I compare what I'm eating to others, and I feel bad if I eat more than they are.
	18. I worry about what people think about my eating.
	19. I eat less food when I'm around other people, regardless of my hunger and fullness level.
	20. I believe that I have to lose weight in order to be healthy.

Dieting Mentality Reflection

Review the diet mentality statements you checked off.

1. Do you see any patterns in your thoughts or behaviors?

    _____

    _____

    _____

    _____

2. How frequently do you have these thoughts or speak them in conversation?

    _____

    _____

    _____

    _____

3. How has maintaining this language kept you in a diet mentality?

    _____

    _____

    _____

    _____

As you begin to practice the principles of Intuitive Eating, these thoughts and behaviors will fade into the background and eventually disappear. Whenever you're feeling bad about what you ate, reflect on what you've just said to yourself—there's a good chance it was some form of dieting mentality. For now, simply labeling these types of thoughts as "diet mentality" is a great step. Because *paying attention*—without judgment—is needed for meaningful change to take place. This is a characteristic of compassion, which plays an important role in the journey of becoming an Intuitive Eater.

Prevent Turning Intuitive Eating into a Diet!

It's important to remember that the process of Intuitive Eating is flexible, not rigid. Intuitive Eating is organized around ten principles, but these are not rules! Chronic dieters have an uncanny knack for turning Intuitive Eating into a dieting mentality, the hallmark of which is characterized by rigidity in thinking, rules, and being judgmental, rather than compassionate. As you work through this book and continue to practice Intuitive Eating, it will become easier to recognize the rigidity of the diet mentality when it creeps into your mind. If you are unsure, you can always come back to the section on dieting mentality.

Wrap-Up

In this chapter, you learned about the importance of cultivating compassion and examined your dieting history and dieting thoughts. You practiced ways to let go of the tools of dieting and the language of dieting. Please keep in mind that we live in a dieting culture, so it is easy to be triggered. Letting go of the diet mentality will be an ongoing practice—remember to be patient with yourself.

In the next chapter, you will learn another way to let go of the diet mentality—by listening and honoring your body's cues of hunger.

CHAPTER 2

Principle Two
Honor Your Hunger

Keep your body biologically fed with adequate energy and carbohydrates. Otherwise, you can trigger a primal drive to overeat. Once you reach the moment of excessive hunger, all intentions of moderate, conscious eating are fleeting and irrelevant. Learning to honor the first biological signal of hunger sets the stage for rebuilding trust with yourself and food.

Hunger is a natural biological cue that lets you know that your body needs sustenance. Nourishing your body is as essential to life as is breathing. Honoring your hunger is an important part of Intuitive Eating. Chronic dieters often deny their biological hunger, only to have it backlash. Their hunger increases and sets off a biological cascade, both physically and psychologically—"primal hunger," an urgent and intense desire to eat—which often results in overeating. Primal hunger is a state that occurs when biological hunger has gone unanswered for far too long. It's akin to holding your breath under water until the need for air is desperate and then finally coming up to the surface. Your first breath after prolonged submersion is primal—a profound, grasping inhalation—rather than a polite intake of breath. It's a compensatory biological reaction.

Here's an example. Let's say you eat lunch at noon and get pulled into an unexpected meeting after work. After work, you finally head out to the gym, later than usual. Your plan for dinner was to eat a meal you often enjoy: pasta with grilled salmon, served with a satisfying salad. But there you are, pounding the treadmill; it's eight at night, and you are so hungry that all you can think of is eating. You grow irritable and impatient. There's a new word that aptly describes this state, *hangry*, a fusion between *hungry* and *angry*.

It becomes difficult to enjoy your workout, which is ordinarily a stress-relieving end to your workday. You can't stand it anymore. You reach for your cell phone and order a pizza topped with grilled chicken, so it will be at your house the moment you get there. As you drive home, you plan to eat a couple of slices with a salad. But instead, you find yourself intensely devouring one slice after another and too full to eat the salad. That is the power of biology.

The term *hunger* technically refers to the biological need to eat, but it often is used to describe the mere *desire* to eat (without the presence of hunger cues). We use the description *biological hunger* as a point of clarity, which refers to the cues originating from your body saying it needs nourishment.

Many of our clients view hunger as the enemy—something to fight off or ignore, or something to be tricked. When experiencing biological hunger, the mind of a chronic dieter will habitually say *Don't*, *It's not time to eat*, or *You can't be hungry yet*. But ignoring hunger and employing trickery—such as drinking water or eating "air food"—makes the process of eating confusing to the body. Air foods are foods that provide volume with little substance or energy, like rice cakes or sugar-free gelatin. When the rules of your mind conflict with the direct experience of your body (hunger cues, which you'll learn about in the activities later in this chapter), it erodes trust in your body, and further confusion ensues. As these hunger cues are disrupted, you can wind up feeling numb, without a sense of what hunger feels like. If your hunger is silenced too often, it can go dormant, making it easier for you to eat for other reasons, which is known as *eating in the absence of hunger*. It's no wonder that many of our clients say, "I just don't know how to eat anymore."

The chronic food deprivation of dieting is a traumatic assault on the body and mind—a nutritional trauma, similar to actual starvation—which needs to be remedied with consistent nourishment. If you also have a history of food scarcity—whether from poverty or childhood neglect—dieting and the act of denying your hunger recreates that trauma. Every meal can feel as if it's the last time you will get to eat, even if you are safe and financially secure.

Honoring your hunger is a key step in healing your relationship with food. But this is not always easy. It can be challenging to honor your hunger if you have been avoiding it or simply not listening for it. Perhaps the signs of hunger from your body have been dormant for a long time.

The activities in this chapter will help you to

- cultivate general body cue awareness;

- identify your attunement disrupters and solutions;

- identify important components of self-care;

- identify the many different signs of hunger;

- identify the various qualities of hunger;

- learn how to rate your hunger; and

- develop a plan for nourishment, as self-care, for times when you are not experiencing hunger, such as when you are sick or experiencing a lot of stress.

Body Cue Awareness: Interoceptive Awareness

Perceiving the physical sensations that arise from within your body is called *interoceptive awareness* or *interoception*. Interoceptive awareness is a powerful and innate ability, which includes perceiving the physical cues of hunger and satiety, bodily states such as a rapid heartbeat and a full bladder, and the physical sensations produced by emotions, like the rush of heat and jitteriness you feel when you panic. This is the *direct experience* of your physical body. Being attuned to these sensations gives you powerful information into your physiological and psychological state, which can help determine what you need to do in order to meet your needs.

It's not surprising that studies have shown that Intuitive Eaters have higher interoceptive awareness (Herbert et al. 2013; Tylka 2006; Tylka and Kroon Van Diest 2013). People who meditate also have higher interoceptive awareness. The principles of Intuitive Eating either cultivate interoceptive awareness or remove the obstacles to that awareness. The obstacles usually originate in your mind—in the form of rules, beliefs, and thoughts. For example, you might have a rule that you can't eat any snacks, only to find yourself very hungry between meals. That's an obstacle and a conflict. Your body is biologically hungry, but your rule is *No eating between meals*. You might try to ignore or trick that hunger, only to find yourself even hungrier and more desperate to eat. We will explore this issue in more depth later in the chapter (in the section I Can't Be Hungry—I Just Ate! Distinguishing Between Thoughts and Hunger Cues).

Can You Perceive Your Heart Rate?

One way that researchers measure people's interoceptive awareness ability is by asking them to perceive their heart beating—to count their heartbeats—without physically touching the body for a pulse. This three-part activity will help you to listen to and connect with your body sensations by placing your attention on your heart rate. Please find a quiet place to sit without distraction for this experiment.

Part 1. Warm-Up: Physically Monitor Your Pulse

If you have participated in physical activities, you might have been taught how to monitor your heart rate by taking your pulse. Using your right hand, place your index and middle finger on the wrist of your left hand and feel the sensation of your pulse or heartbeat. It's important to be patient. Once you can feel your pulse, count your heartbeats for one minute. Do this a couple of times, until you feel comfortable locating your pulse.

Part 2. Perceive Your Heart Rate

It's imperative that there is no distraction when you do this activity. This exercise requires gentleness and patience. Place your hands, palms down, comfortably on your legs (this is just a resting spot for your hands). Breathing normally, take a few relaxing breaths. When you feel calm and relaxed, place your attention on your heart beating. Without manually finding a pulse, silently count each heartbeat in your body for one minute. This will take some practice; not everybody can sense their heartbeat on the first try.

Part 3. Reflection

Take a moment to reflect on the following questions and write your responses.

1. Were you able to perceive the sensation of your heart beating? If yes, go to question 2. If no, skip to question 3.

   _____

   _____

2. Where in your body did you perceive your heart beating? (It's possible to experience it in many different places, such as your hands or your chest.) Did you perceive your heart beating in more than one location in your body?

   _____

   _____

   _____

3. What was your self-talk like when you were trying to perceive your heart beating? Were your thoughts critical and harsh? Or perhaps your thoughts were kind and compassionate?

   _____

   _____

   _____

Simply perceiving your own heart rate is one of many ways to practice attunement. For people who have body dissatisfaction and anxiety around eating, this is a novel way to connect with their body, because it is about purely listening. A meditation practice is another way to connect with your body. In many meditation practices, your attention is simply placed on the experience of your breathing. As with perceiving for your heartbeat, it is simply a practice of listening to your body.

Suggestion: try to set aside five minutes a day to practice perceiving your heart rate. (You are obviously alive, with a beating heart—this is just a new level of listening, which will get easier with practice.)

Getting to Know Your Body's Physical Sensations

Let's explore *where* in your body you experience different physical states or emotions, such as sleepiness or stress, and where you feel different biological cues, such as a full bladder or feeling thirst. In this section, we'll also explore the quality of these physical sensations. For example, if you are relaxed and a bit sleepy, your sleepiness might feel pleasant. If, on the other hand, you are jet-lagged and chronically sleep deprived, it may feel unpleasant—to say the least!

Paying attention to your body's physical sensations on a regular basis will help you learn to hear your hunger sensations. Listening to different body sensations is a form of cross-training for body cue awareness.

Please keep in mind that these body sensations are not "right" or "wrong"—they are just information. If you are not used to connecting with and listening to your body, just provide your best guesses in the following activity.

The purpose of this exercise is to help increase your awareness of physical sensations that arise from your biological cues and body states. This exercise will take a few days to fully complete. The left-hand column lists a series of body cues and body states. For each, reflect upon where in your body you may experience a physical sensation related to that cue and place an X in the corresponding column: head, eyes, and so forth. For example, when you are thirsty, you might feel the sensation in your mouth. Next, in the last three columns on the right, reflect on the overall experience—is it pleasant, unpleasant, or neutral? For example, when you are thirsty, is the sensation pleasant, unpleasant, or neutral? (Whether the sensation is pleasant, unpleasant, or neutral might depend on its intensity. Thirst might usually be neutral, but unpleasant if it is extreme. For this exercise, don't worry about this detail—why a body cue feels one way or another. The point of this exercise is simply to help you learn to recognize the sensations themselves.)

Getting to Know Your Body: Physical Sensations from Biological Cues and Body States

	Head	Eyes	Mouth	Neck or Throat	Shoulders	Chest	Stomach	Bladder	Legs	Overall Pleasant	Overall Unpleasant	Overall Neutral
Body Cues												
Thirsty												
Need to Urinate												
Hungry												
Full												
Body State												
Sleepy												
Restless												
Sick or Ill												
Rested												
Stress												

ATTUNEMENT REFLECTION

1. When they first try to become familiar with various body sensations, some people have difficulty noticing them until the experience is intense or unpleasant. Was this true for you?

_____

_____

_____

2. Did you notice any patterns or trends about your body sensations? Did anything surprise you?

_____

_____

_____

As you practice paying attention to your body wisdom, you will gradually develop a heightened awareness of a variety of sensations, which will give you powerful information for your physical and emotional well-being.

Self-Care and Attunement Disrupters

An attunement disrupter is anything that interferes with your ability to hear and respond to the needs of your body in a timely manner. Disrupters include distractions, thoughts, rules, beliefs, and a lack of self-care.

What do you do to take care of yourself? That is, what do you actively do to get your basic needs met and to manage stress? We ask this important question because it can be difficult to hear your body cues like hunger, let alone respond to them in a timely manner, if you are living a demanding and chaotic lifestyle. Adequate self-care is a critical foundation to Intuitive Eating. When you are in the throes of stress, whether it's fighting deadlines or chasing toddlers in diapers, your body's biological fight-or-flight survival system is activated. Your blood flow is diverted away from your digestive system and shunted to your extremities to help you flee or fight the enemy—resulting in a lack of hunger cues. (Biologically, using energy to digest the food in the stomach will just slow you down if you are trying to outrun a tiger).

Thanks to technology, life seems to be "on" 24/7 these days, and it's all too easy to get swept away, juggling too many projects and obligations. If you are chronically sleep deprived— whether it's from stress or just because you have trouble getting yourself to bed on time, because you are posting on social media—it can affect your ability to hear your hunger or fullness cues. Unless you have boundaries to protect your precious time and energy, you can find yourself chronically zapped and depleted—both emotionally and physically exhausted.

Contrary to popular belief, self-care is not just about getting massages and taking bubble baths, though those activities could certainly be considered a form of self-care. *Self-care* is defined as the daily process of attending to your basic physical and emotional needs, which include the shaping of your daily routine, relationships, and environment, as needed to promote self-care (Cook-Cottone 2015). It includes a broad range of activities, such as getting enough sleep and attending to emotional, physical, relationship, and spiritual needs. Such activities should not be viewed as a luxury or a selfish pursuit. In fact, self-care is so important that the American Psychological Association has included it as an ethical imperative for psychologists—so they will be emotionally and mentally stable enough to help their patients (Barnett et al. 2007).

In this section, we will explore self-care activities and attunement disrupters. In the following chart, please check the boxes that apply to you. Notice that in the top half of each category, there are positive behaviors which serve your self-care; in the bottom half of the chart, there are attunement disrupters that work against your taking care of your needs. Keep in mind that this chart is by no means all-inclusive.

Self-Care Assessment

	Physical	Emotional and Psychological	Relationships
Positive Behaviors	☐ I get enough sleep to feel rested and restored when I wake up. ☐ I get regular medical and dental checkups. ☐ I take time off work or school when I am sick. ☐ I wear clothes that I like and that feel comfortable. ☐ I take vacations. ☐ I engage in a physical activity that I enjoy at least five times a week. ☐ Other	☐ I make time for self-reflection. ☐ I am aware of my thoughts, without judgment. ☐ I am aware of my feelings, without judgment. ☐ I write in a journal. ☐ I identify comforting activities and places and seek them out. ☐ I make time to relax. ☐ I make time to play. ☐ I find things that make me laugh. ☐ I have hobbies and interests outside of work or school. ☐ I have compassion for myself and others. ☐ I seek therapy when needed. ☐ Other	☐ I spend time with people whom I enjoy and who sustain and support me. ☐ I have someone in my life who would listen to me if I were upset or just needed to talk (friends, family, a therapist, or clergy). ☐ I stay in contact with important people in my life. ☐ I make time to spend with my family. ☐ Other

	Physical	Emotional and Psychological	Relationships
Attunement Disrupters	☐ I often skip meals when I am pressed for time.	☐ I feel guilty if I am not productive or doing something important.	☐ I don't like to burden my friends or family with my problems.
	☐ I watch more than two hours of television a day.	☐ I do not know how to relax.	☐ My family doesn't support me when I have problems.
	☐ I exercise too much, such as when I am sick or injured.	☐ I engage in harsh or critical self-talk.	☐ I worry about what people think of me.
	☐ I smoke (or vape).	☐ I don't allow myself to feel my feelings or cry.	☐ I withdraw from people when I am stressed out.
	☐ I go long periods of time without eating.	☐ I have a difficult time managing stress.	☐ Other
	☐ I overeat or undereat when I am stressed.	☐ I self-silence my thoughts and feelings.	
	☐ I often multitask while I eat, watching television, checking e-mail, or reading.	☐ My life feels out of control.	
	☐ I am often sleep deprived.	☐ Other	
	☐ I drink more than the recommended levels of alcohol (more than one or two drinks per day).		
	☐ Other		

	Spiritual	Boundaries
Positive Behaviors	☐ I spend time in nature. ☐ I make time for reflection. ☐ I seek or participate in a spiritual connection or community. ☐ I am aware of nonmaterial aspects of life. ☐ I seek experiences of awe. ☐ I have a meditation practice. ☐ I pray. ☐ I read or study inspirational books or articles. ☐ Other	☐ I maintain a manageable schedule at work or school, which includes taking breaks. ☐ I take breaks from electronic media including my computer, smartphone, or television. ☐ I say no to extra projects or responsibilities if I am overscheduled. ☐ I set limits with my family and friends. ☐ I set limits with volunteer projects. ☐ I set limits with work, such as not working while on vacation. ☐ I strive for balance among work, family, school, play, relationships, and rest. ☐ I speak up when others attempt to cross my boundaries. ☐ Other
Attunement Disrupters	☐ I am mainly drawn to material things. ☐ I don't take any time to reflect on the meaning of my life. ☐ I always believe that I don't have enough. ☐ I don't consider the things in my life for which I am grateful. ☐ I don't consider that I actually have a purpose in this life. ☐ Other	☐ I have a hard time saying no to people's requests. ☐ I feel the need to make others happy. ☐ I feel selfish if I say no to a request. ☐ I tend to take on too many projects and activities. ☐ I automatically say yes to requests, without reflecting on my schedule or prior commitments. ☐ I take pride in being super busy. ☐ Other

SELF-CARE REFLECTION

Using the information from your Self-Care Assessment, answer the following questions.

1. What trends did you notice in your positive self-care behaviors?

    _____

    _____

    _____

2. What are your strengths in self-care behaviors?

    _____

    _____

    _____

3. Are there any categories of self-care that you have not been currently addressing?

    _____

    _____

    _____

4. What categories of self-care need more attention or perhaps just consistency?

    _____

    _____

    _____

5. What were your attunement disrupters?

    _____

    _____

    _____

Self-Care Practices to Increase

Review each of the self-care categories from your assessment. Describe one or two strategies that you are willing to consistently implement to improve your self-care.

Physical

Example: I will work on consistently getting enough sleep by getting to bed, with lights out, by ten thirty.

_____

_____

_____

Emotional and Psychological

Example: I will spend thirty minutes relaxing when I get home from work.

_____

_____

_____

Boundaries

Example: I will politely decline new volunteer projects until I finish my current commitment of volunteering at my son's school.

_____

_____

_____

Spiritual

Example: I will start meditating for ten minutes a day, in the morning.

_____

_____

_____

Relationships

Example: I will reach out by phone to at least one of my good friends once a week.

_____

_____

_____

Attunement Disrupters to Decrease

Review each of the attunement distractor categories from your assessment. Describe one or two issues on which you are willing to work.

Physical

Example: I often eat while multitasking. I will eat at least one meal a day without distraction.

_____

_____

_____

Emotional and Psychological

Example: I do not know how to relax. I will give myself permission to relax by reading something fun, unrelated to work or school, at least five times per week.

_____

_____

_____

Boundaries

Example: I automatically say yes to requests, without considering my own schedule and commitments. I will practice delaying my response to requests by saying something like, "I need to check my schedule, and I will get back to you tomorrow to let you know if I am able to help you." This will allow me to think carefully before saying yes or no.

_____

_____

_____

Spiritual

Example: I have no spiritual practice. I will read one inspirational article each week.

_____

_____

_____

Relationships

Example: I frequently isolate myself when I am stressed. I will accept at least one invitation per week in order to be social.

_____

_____

_____

Getting to Know Your Biological Hunger

Biological hunger may be experienced in a variety of ways, with different sensations in different parts of your body. It can vary from person to person. There are also different qualities to the experience of hunger. For example, if you get too hungry (as in ravenous), it's generally an unpleasant experience, but if you are mildly hungry, it will often be pleasant.

Reflection

Think about a recent time when you got too hungry. Perhaps you had to stay late after work or school and didn't have a chance to eat dinner until eight hours after lunch. What was the intensity of your hunger like? What was the quality of the experience like for you: pleasant, unpleasant, or neutral? Where did you feel it in the body?

_____

_____

_____

Hunger-Body-Mind Connection

When your body is hungry, it tries to get your attention in a variety of ways, from mood and energy changes to increased thoughts about food. The longer you wait to nourish your body, the more intense these experiences will be. Getting to know your hunger cues might seem frustrating, especially if you have not experienced hunger in a long time—perhaps because you've been numb from stress or perhaps you don't let yourself get hungry at all. The more you listen to your body, the more you will begin to hear and experience the subtler signs of hunger.

Keep in mind that everyone is different, and there is no right or wrong way to experience hunger. Here are some of the different ways that you may experience signs of hunger. Check off those that you experience.

- ☐ Stomach: A variety of sensations including rumbling, gurgling, gnawing, or emptiness. While this is a common way of experiencing hunger, there are many people who do not experience hunger signs in their stomach.

- ☐ Throat and esophagus: Dull ache, gnawing.

- ☐ Head: Cloudy thinking, light-headedness, headache, difficulty focusing and concentrating. Experiencing more thoughts about food and eating.

- ☐ Mood: Irritability or crankiness. Perhaps you have to work harder to refrain from snapping, even though you don't present as irritable to the outside world.

- ☐ Energy: Waning, perhaps even to the point of sleepiness. There can be dullness and even apathy toward doing anything.

- ☐ Numbness: Overall lethargy.

- ☐ Other: _____

Getting to Know Your Hunger

To get in touch with the nuances of your hunger, it helps to check in many times throughout the day. A handy way to do this is by using a rating scale from 0 to 10, where 0 is painful hunger and 10 is painful fullness. Many researchers use a rating system like this when they are evaluating hunger and fullness issues (which is known as a *visual analogue rating*). This type of rating is also used for pain, when you are admitted to the hospital, because like hunger, pain is a subjective feeling. That's why there is no right or wrong number, this is merely a method that helps you listen and become attuned to your hunger cues. The following chart gives qualitative descriptions of the 0 to 10 scale in more detail.

	Rating	Description of Hunger and Fullness Sensations	Overall Quality of Sensation		
			Pleasant	Unpleasant	Neutral
Over Hungry	0	Painfully hungry. This is primal hunger, which is very intense and urgent.		X	
	1	Ravenous and irritable. Anxious to eat.		X	
	2	Very hungry. Looking forward to a hearty meal or snack.	X		
Normal Eating Range	3	Hungry and ready to eat, but without urgency. It's a polite hunger.	X		
	4	Subtly hungry, slightly empty.			X
	5	Neutral. Neither hungry nor full.			X
	6	Beginning to feel emerging fullness.			X
	7	Comfortable fullness. You feel satisfied and content.	X		
Over Full	8	A little too full. This doesn't feel pleasant, but it has not quite emerged into an unpleasant experience.			X
	9	Very full, too full. You feel uncomfortable, as if you need to unbutton your pants or remove your belt.		X	
	10	Painfully full, stuffed. You may feel nauseous.		X	

REFLECTION

Review the chart on Description of Hunger and Fullness Sensations. Reflect on your usual hunger states and answer the following questions to the best of your ability. (It's okay if you don't know. The next exercise will give you plenty of opportunity to practice).

1. At which rating do you usually *feel* the sensations of hunger? Perhaps 0, perhaps 2?

_____

_____

_____

2. By the time you honor your hunger, does your hunger experience tend to be pleasant, unpleasant, or neutral?

_____

_____

_____

Hunger Discovery Scale

In order to really get dialed in to the nuances of your hunger, you will need repeated listening and experience. It's no different than learning to play a musical instrument—without practice, your ability will not improve.

Using the Hunger Discovery Scale Journal on the next page, keep track of your hunger rating, the quality of your hunger, and the foods eaten for a meal or snack. Do try to be accurate with the time that you ate, as it will help you see any patterns and trends in the intensity of hunger between meals. Do this for several days. (You may want to make copies of the Hunger Discovery Scale Journal.)

First, note the time and rate your hunger by circling the number that best reflects your hunger level before your meal or snack (based on the hunger and fullness discovery scale above, with 0 being primal hunger and 10 being stuffed to the gills). Next, take note of the quality of your hunger. Is it pleasant, unpleasant, or neutral? Place a check in the box that applies to you.

Hunger Discovery Scale Journal

Time	Hunger Rating (0-10)	Quality of Hunger			Meal/Food Eaten	Comments
		Pleasant	Unpleasant	Neutral		

HUNGER DISCOVERY SCALE REFLECTION

After you have completed the Hunger Discovery Scale Journal for several days, answer the following questions.

1. What trends do you notice with your hunger rating?

_____

_____

_____

2. At which level does the sensation of hunger feel just right for you? Perhaps a rating of 2 or 3?

_____

_____

_____

3. What pattern of eating, in regards to timing, works best for you? Perhaps you feel best eating at least every four to five hours or every two to three hours?

_____

_____

_____

4. If you ate lighter or smaller meals or snacks, how did that affect the frequency of your hunger? For example, does your hunger emerge sooner for the next meal or snack? Perhaps it feels like you are always eating?

_____

_____

_____

Nourishment as Self-Care

If you are under chronic stress or have an illness, you really can't rely on hunger cues to adequately nourish your body. This can also be the case if you are an athlete undergoing intense training—hunger is temporary blunted for a couple of hours. These conditions are usually temporary, but your body still needs nourishment. This is like having a broken gas gauge on your car which always indicates a full gas tank. It might say it is full, but you still need to put gas in your tank. Your rational mind overrides the gas gauge indicator. You must make note of how far you drive and get gas when you know you are running low. Similarly, if you do not experience hunger cues, you will need to call upon your rational thought to keep yourself nourished. (Remember, Intuitive Eating is a dynamic interplay of instinct, emotion, and rational thought). This might seem like it goes against the Intuitive Eating protocol of listening to your body, but in situations where your hunger cues are offline, it is really a type of self-care in the form of nourishment.

It's helpful to have a self-care plan for eating during these phases of duress. If you are an athlete, it might mean having several self-care meals throughout the day. If you are under chronic stress, it may mean that you need to do this for several days or weeks (or as long as you need). It's much easier to plan ahead for this when you are feeling well, rather than waiting until you are under the gun. Here are some general guidelines:

1. The foods and meals you eat need to be adequate in energy to sustain your body.

2. It's generally best not to go longer than four to five hours without eating. (That's how long you can generally maintain your blood sugar at a normal level during waking hours, depending on how much you ate and the composition of what you ate at the previous meal. Some people, however, feel true hunger signals after three to four hours without eating).

3. It's best that what you plan to prepare also matches your energy level at the time. For example, if you are drained and exhausted, you will not likely want to cook an elaborate meal, even if you usually enjoy cooking.

4. A general pattern of eating that works is to have at least three meals and a morning and afternoon snack. (This is only a suggestion, not a mandate).

My Self-Care Nourishment Plan: Nutrition 911

Create your Nutrition 911 plan for self-care nourishment by creating a list of what you could eat when your hunger cues are simply not present and you have little desire to eat. Remember, this is not a rigid meal plan—it's simply an opportunity to provide examples of emergency meals and snacks that you might enjoy—or at least tolerate—in order to fuel your body.

1. Reflect on meals that are easy for you to prepare (or pick up), that are appealing, and that usually sustain your body for a few hours. List these meals in the Meal Ideas column.

2. Sometimes when you are incredibly stressed, eating a meal might seem like an impossible task. In these situations, you might feel better eating smaller meals (or even just snacks) more frequently throughout the day. Reflect on snacks or light meals that usually sustain you for a couple of hours, and list them in the Snack Ideas column.

As you generate these ideas, it's important to be flexible and adjust as needed. You won't really know if your ideas work until you test them out under real-life conditions, when you have little desire to eat. But through testing out your ideas, you will learn which Nutrition 911 meals or snacks are effective for you.

Meal Ideas	Snack Ideas

I Can't Be Hungry—I Just Ate! Distinguishing Between Thoughts and Hunger Cues

Sometimes there is confusion about whether or not to eat, because thoughts may interfere with the direct experience of hunger cues from your body. Here's a common scenario we hear over and over again: Let's say you ate breakfast at seven this morning. Yet just one hour later, at eight, you are clearly biologically hungry. Your stomach is gnawing and growling. You feel empty and have a desire to eat. But your first thought is, *I can't be hungry—I just ate!* And then you try to distract yourself from your hunger and wait it out until lunch. It's understandable to feel puzzled or even annoyed that you are experiencing hunger so soon after eating a meal. Yet there are a number of reason why your body might simply need more nourishment:

- The day before, you had an unusually higher level of physical activity.

- You ate markedly less the day before.

- Your breakfast at seven might, in actuality, have been more of a snack than a meal.

- You are just having a hungrier day.

- You worked out early that morning, so your hunger was somewhat blunted when you sat down for breakfast, and you didn't eat enough.

- You have a physical condition, such as being premenstrual, which is making you hungrier than usual.

Honoring hunger in a timely manner can sometimes be inconvenient and confusing, but it is really no different then needing to take a bathroom break even though you went just an hour ago. These are both basic biological cues—the only difference is that people don't usually feel guilty or believe they did something wrong if they need another trip to the bathroom. It's just a bit annoying, not a moral indictment.

Every time you experience biological hunger and you respond by honoring that hunger with nourishment, you build trust and connection with your body. Every time you honor hunger because your here-and-now body is hungry, you will get clarity, not confusion.

The next activity will help you explore the differences between hunger cues and thoughts, to help you clarify what you would need in order to take care of your body. In the Mind, Body Cue, or Self-Care Worksheet, read each statement and then place a check mark in the appropriate box to indicate which category fits the statement best. Some statements may fit into more than one category, but each one will fit best into one of them:

- *Mind* reflects a thought, opinion, or judgment.

- *Body Cue* reflects a direct experience or sensation from your body.

- *Self-Care* is an action that takes care of your needs, but will also involve the mind.

Mind, Body Cue, or Self-Care Worksheet

Statement	Category		
	Mind	Body Cue	Self-Care
1. I can't be hungry—I just ate breakfast one hour ago.			
2. I deserve to eat this food, because I worked out at the gym today.			
3. My stomach feels empty, and I'm having difficulty concentrating. I need to eat.			
4. I skip breakfast, which will keep me from feeling hungrier the rest of the day.			
5. I am afraid that if I eat this snack to honor my hunger, it will add unnecessary calories.			
6. I did not exercise today, but I ate a lot of calories! It was way too many calories, considering I didn't even work out, but I was hungry all day, so I ate.			
7. I haven't eaten since breakfast, about six hours ago; therefore, I should eat something, even though I don't feel hungry.			
8. I don't know when we will arrive at my parents' house for dinner. It's a long drive. I'd better pack a snack.			
9. I'm anxious about my presentation, my mouth is dry, and my stomach is queasy—therefore, I'm going to skip breakfast.			
10. I don't feel very hungry for dinner. I will eat something light but satisfying.			

Worksheet Answers and Explanation: Mind, Body Cue, or Self-Care?

Statement	Category		
	Mind	Body Cue	Self-Care
1. I can't be hungry—I just ate breakfast one hour ago. *This is a thought (mind). What is your here-and-now body experiencing, physically?*			
2. I deserve to eat this food, because I worked out at the gym today. *This is a thought (mind). This thought might reflect a reward or entitlement.*			
3. My stomach feels empty and I'm having difficulty concentrating. I need to eat. *This is an experience from your body. The statement is also a thought, an assessment, which reflects the need to eat, which could also be self-care.*			
4. I skip breakfast, which will keep me from feeling hungrier the rest of the day. *This is a thought (mind), which also reflects the dieting mentality.*			
5. I am afraid that if I eat this snack to honor my hunger, it will add unnecessary calories. *This is a thought (mind), which also reflects the dieting mentality.*			

Statement	Category		
	Mind	Body Cue	Self-Care
6. I did not exercise today and ate a lot of calories! I feel like that is way too many calories because I didn't work out. But I was hungry all day, so I ate. *This is a thought (mind), reflecting the dieting mentality. But the direct experience of the body was that hunger was honored. This is a good example of a shift toward honoring hunger rather than obeying the judgmental thought. Thoughts tend to gradually fade away rather than suddenly disappear.*			
7. I haven't eaten since breakfast, about six hours ago; therefore, I should eat something, even though I don't feel hungry. *Notice that self-care comes from the thought (mind) How do you distinguish a self-care thought?*			
8. I don't know when we will arrive at my parents' house for dinner. It's a long drive. I'd better pack a snack. *This is a self-care thought.*			
9. I'm anxious about my presentation, my mouth is dry, and my stomach is queasy—therefore, I'm going to skip breakfast. *The sensations are a direct experience of the body associated with anxiety, which is masking the biological need for nourishment. The self-care act would be to eat something that would not amplify the nausea.*			
10. I don't feel very hungry for dinner. I will eat something light, but satisfying. *This question is ambiguous for the sake of prompting inquiry. How might this statement reflect the direct experience of your body? Is making a plan to eat something light a form of dieting or self-care?*			

REFLECTION

1. How can you distinguish between a dieting-mentality thought and a thought that will serve your best interest—a thought reflecting self-care?

_____

_____

_____

2. How can awareness of your thoughts, compared with being aware of the direct experience from your body cues, help you become an Intuitive Eater?

_____

_____

_____

Wrap-Up

You now have the basic practices to become aware of and to honor your hunger. Keep in mind that knowledge and practice are not the same thing. It will be important for you to maintain an ongoing practice of identifying and responding to your hunger. For some people, it may take a few weeks to really recognize the nuances of hunger. For others, it can take months. Everybody is different. There is no correct timetable or deadline to accomplish this principle. Remember to be patient; be kind to yourself in this process. In the next chapter, you will learn how to make peace with food.

CHAPTER 3

Principle Three
Make Peace with Food

Call a truce—stop the food fight! Give yourself unconditional permission to eat. If you tell yourself that you can't or shouldn't have a particular food, it can lead to intense feelings of deprivation that build into uncontrollable cravings and, often, bingeing. When you finally give in to your forbidden food, eating will be experienced with such intensity that it usually results in Last Supper overeating and overwhelming guilt.

You can't make peace with your eating by declaring a war on your body or the foods you put into it. Forbidding yourself specific foods can have a paradoxical rebound effect that triggers overeating. You have already seen how biological deprivation (hunger) can lead to overeating. But there's also another powerful factor at play—the psychological effects of deprivation—which uncannily fuels obsessive thinking about food, ultimately leading to overeating and disconnection from your body.

Making peace with food is a critical component of Intuitive Eating, which involves eating the food you desire with attunement to your hunger and fullness levels. It is the process of making your food choices *emotionally* equal, without placing shame or judgment on them, whether you are eating green jelly beans or a piece of broccoli. Your dignity remains intact, regardless of your food choices. You are not a bad or good person based on what you eat!

When you truly give yourself permission to eat what you like, it allows you to really experience the taste and the effect of the food in your body. If the food is not off-limits, the threat of the now-or-never type of overeating is gone. When you no longer feel you are depriving yourself of a food, it gives you the space that allows you to ask, *Do I really like the taste of this food? Do I like how this food feels in my body? Would I choose to feel this way again after eating this meal or snack? Would I choose to eat in this manner again?* After all, this will not be the last time you eat this food—so why would you want to eat it in a way that does not feel good or is not satisfying?

Another purpose of the unconditional permission to eat is to quell the deprivation backlash, which builds with each new diet you try, with yet another food foisted onto the do-not-eat list. Ultimately, this principle is about valuing your emotional health and taking morality out of your eating, all while increasing the flexibility of your food choices.

In this chapter, we will briefly explore the science and psychology behind this principle and what it really means to eat with unconditional permission. The activities here will help you to

- explore your readiness to make peace with eating any food;

- learn how to create a safe environment to make peace with food;

- practice how to select a specific food for experimentation; and

- learn how to assess and check in with the eating experience.

Why Unconditional Permission to Eat Is Vital: The Deprivation Set-Up

Any time you are deprived of something you like or need, you begin to long for it—whether it's a longing for a shower after days of camping or a craving for fresh fruit and vegetables while traveling through a developing country. The deprivation effect is profound in dieters.

In order to control their eating, chronic dieters abide by rigid rules that dictate what they can and cannot eat, with little regard to their experience of hunger, fullness, and satisfaction. Consequently, chronic dieters live in their heads and second-guess the needs of their bodies. After a while, interoceptive awareness (the ability to perceive physical sensations that arise from within the body) goes dormant. Living and eating by the rules seems to work just fine, until something goes awry. That something could be an event, an emotion, a thought, a craving, or just sheer hunger that triggers the violation of a sacred food rule. Just a bite of the wrong food at the wrong time, and all bets are off. Bye-bye food rules. All restraint is broken, and an all-or-none food feast ensues—for tomorrow a new day begins, and the forbidden foods will be off-limits, once again. Better hurry and eat it now, before you change your mind. We even see this phenomenon in people who are getting ready to *start* a diet. Here's a brief look at the fascinating factors that drive this all-or-none pattern of eating, in which food restriction contributes to overconsumption.

Dietary Restraint Theory

Dietary restraint theory describes what happens when fastidious dieters go off their diet or break their food rules. Canadian researchers Janet Polivy and C. Peter Herman pioneered the restraint theory based on observing a predictable eating pattern among dieters. Their research is a key influence in the Intuitive Eating model (Tribole and Resch 1995, 2012).

THE WHAT-THE-HELL EFFECT

Dieters tend to evaluate their successes or failures of eating in terms of the current day. Success requires getting through the day with no violations of the diet. Even just thinking that you have blown your diet is enough to trigger the consumption of more food, regardless of hunger or fullness levels. They aptly described this restraint-overeating cycle as the *what-the-hell effect* (Herman and Polivy 1984).

PERCEPTION

Restrained eaters are likely to overeat even if they only *perceived* that they violated one of their food rules. Many dieters have rules about not eating high-calorie foods, so the researchers set up a sneaky taste-testing study. Dieters were told they would be sampling a high-calorie food (when in actuality, it was not!). The mere perception of blowing their diet was enough to trigger overeating (Urbszat, Herman, and Polivy 2002).

ANTICIPATION OF FOOD RESTRICTION

A study of chocolate lovers found that when a chocolate restriction was imposed for three weeks, it triggered an increase in their chocolate consumption before and after the restriction period (Keeler, Mattes, and Tan 2015). For many dieters, just the anticipation of starting a new diet is enough to trigger overeating—a farewell-to-food feast.

Consequently, restrained eaters do not really end up eating less food overall. Researchers suggest that a high restraint eating score (meaning a high degree of restrained eating) seems to more accurately reflect eating-related guilt rather than actual food consumed (de Witt Huberts, Evers, and de Ridder 2013).

THE IRONY OF THOUGHT SUPPRESSION

A large body of research indicates that thought suppression is ineffective. Moreover, it can be counterproductive, helping to assure the very state of mind one had hoped to avoid (Wenzlaff and Wegner 2000). Imagine being told, "Don't think of a white bear." This is an example of thought suppression. Give it a try—close your eyes for a minute and try not to think of a white bear. What did you discover?

Similarly, in a seminal study, researchers asked people to think aloud in a stream-of-consciousness manner while trying not to think of a white bear (Wegner et al. 1987). This innocuous instruction triggered a rebound effect, and the bear was mentioned at least once a minute! Furthermore, the don't-think-of-a-white-bear group had more thoughts of this furry Nordic mammal than the comparison group, which had been given the opposite instruction—to think about a white bear. Research has similarly shown that trying to suppress food-related thoughts not only increases thinking about the food but may also increase eating behavior (Barnes and Tantleff-Dunn 2010).

THE FORBIDDEN-FRUIT PHENOMENON

Don't eat the red food. The allure of a forbidden food is heightened in non-dieters as well. In a clever study design, a group of children was told that they could not eat the red M&M candies, but they could eat as many of the yellow M&M's as they wanted (same candy, just a different color). Guess which candy got the most attention and consumption? Yes, the red ones (Jansen, Mulkens, and Jansen 2007). A similar study found that when kids were not allowed to eat fruit *or* sweets, it led to an increased consumption of both of these foods (Jansen et al. 2008).

A body of research on children has shown that the more a parent restricts his or her child's eating, the more it creates a rebound effect, causing the child to eat more of the forbidden food and to become more disconnected from his or her body. This leads to eating in the absence of hunger and overeating. That child is more likely to grow up with an increased risk of emotional eating and higher BMI, especially for women (Galloway, Farrow, and Martz 2010).

Inventory: What Foods Do You Currently Forbid or Restrict?

This activity is intended to help you picture clearly the impact of having forbidden or restricted foods. Using the worksheet below, list the foods that are currently off-limits. This worksheet is organized by category of foods for the sake of jogging your memory.

Category	Food		
Grains			
Fruits			
Sweets and Desserts			
Processed Foods			
Fats and Fatty Foods			
High-Calorie Foods			
Other			

REFLECTION: YOUR FORBIDDEN FOOD INVENTORY

Review your list and reflect upon the last time you ate one of these foods.

1. Describe your thoughts and eating behavior when you decide to eat one of your forbidden foods.

    _____

    _____

2. While you are eating your forbidden food, are you connected to the taste and your body sensations of emerging fullness? Or would you describe the eating as disconnected, perhaps urgent?

    _____

    _____

3. How does eating one of your forbidden foods affect:

    A. Your eating for the rest of the day?

    _____

    _____

    B. Your mood?

    _____

    _____

    C. How you feel about yourself?

    _____

    _____

Habituation: Familiarity and Exposure Breeds Ordinariness

Forbidden foods remain exciting and novel for dieters, because those foods are not subject to the habituation effect. Habituation explains what happens when you are repeatedly exposed to the same stimulus—whether it's a car, relationship, or food. The novelty of it begins to wear off. For example, the first time you hear your significant other whisper, "I love you," it is quite thrilling. But ten years later, hearing the same "I love you" from the same person, while lovely, is not as exciting.

In the case of eating, habituation is the reason why leftovers become less appealing over time, even if it is your favorite food. The more you eat the same food, the less enticement it offers. It is just food. Sure, it still tastes good, but it becomes no big deal. Several studies have demonstrated the habituation effect with many different foods, including pizza, chocolate, and potato chips (Epstein et al. 2009).

DIETING IMPEDES THE HABITUATION EFFECT

The problem for chronic dieters is that forbidden-food rules prevent the habituation response. Instead, a vicious cycle ensues with each diet: the diet begins with food restriction, followed by broken restraint and the consumption of forbidden foods, which triggers feelings of guilt and a lack of control over eating those foods. That guilt and uncontrolled eating provides false evidence that more rules are needed to constrain the eating. Back to another diet (see fig. 3.1)! The habituation and restraint effect, combined with the forbidden-fruit phenomenon, creates the conditions for a perfect storm of *overeating* forbidden foods. It is no wonder that a growing body of research shows that the more someone diets, the more likely he or she is to engage in binge eating (Holmes et al. 2014).

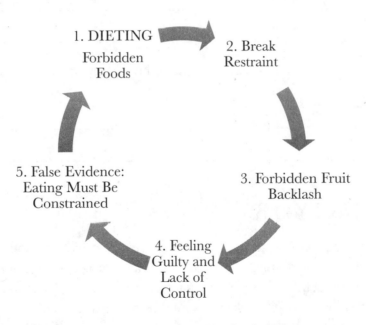

Figure 3.1.   Dieting impedes habituation.

There are two other key factors that can interfere with the habituation effect: distraction and stress. This is a double whammy for dieters. Dieting itself increases the stress response by triggering the body to make more of the stress hormone cortisol (Tomiyama et al. 2010). Eating while distracted disrupts habituation to the rewarding qualities of eating a particular food (Robinson et al. 2013), which means it might take more food to feel satisfied. It is yet another reason why it is so important to eat without distraction as often as you can.

REFLECTION: YOUR "LAST SUPPER" EATING HISTORY

You have just read about the powerful impact of deprivation, dietary restraint, and habituation—now let's examine its impact on your own dieting history. It might be helpful to reflect on the answers from your Dieting History Worksheet in chapter 1.

1. How often do you engage in a farewell-to-food feast to get ready to start a new diet or cleanse routine—rarely, sometimes, or often? Describe this ritual.

   _____

   _____

2. If you perceived that you blew your diet, what behaviors would that trigger: overeating, disregard of your eating for the remainder of the day, or something else? Describe.

   _____

   _____

3. If you have finished your diet or eating program, how likely are you to stay connected to physical sensations of hunger and fullness? Describe.

   _____

   _____

Fears That Hold You Back

In spite of the compelling research, the idea of eating a forbidden food may seem like a threatening proposition. Yet making peace with food is a key principle in improving your relationship with food. If you believe that you are not supposed to eat a particular food at all, why would you stop eating it once you've broken the rule? Instead, eating remains scary, a push-pull struggle with a chronic niggling anxiety every time you eat, especially when forbidden foods are brimming around you. No peace. No freedom. Let's take a closer look at some possible fears.

WHAT ARE YOUR FEARS?

Here is a list of some common fears that might make you feel reluctant to give yourself permission to eat off-limit foods. Check off the statements that apply to you.

Yes	Statement
	1. Once I start eating a forbidden food, I won't stop.
	2. I've tried it before, but it didn't work.
	3. I won't eat healthfully.
	4. I think that I am addicted to my forbidden foods.
	5. I don't trust myself around food.
	6. My friends or family will criticize my food choices.
	7. I don't deserve to eat these foods until I lose weight.
	8. Other

REFLECTION: FEARS ABOUT EATING FORBIDDEN FOOD

As you reflect on these statements and your responses, it's important to keep a self-compassionate perspective. This activity is about discovery and learning, not an exercise in passing judgment on yourself.

1. *I won't stop eating a particular food.* This is a common fear expressed by dieters, which reflects deprivation and a lack of habituation. With no habituation experience, foods like chocolate remain exciting and daunting. Making peace with food is about experiencing habituation. It's understandable that if you have not experienced the ordinariness of a favorite food, you will be reluctant to eat it. When you know that a food is no longer off-limits, you will discover that when you eat past satisfaction, the pleasurable taste of food diminishes, and the physical discomfort from eating too much will become apparent. You'll come to recognize that overeating your favorite foods is no longer worth it. What do you think would happen if you ate your forbidden food every day, at every meal? Would that be a satisfying experience everyday?

_____

_____

2. *I tried eating forbidden foods before, but it didn't work.* You might have behaviorally allowed yourself the freedom to eat forbidden foods, but did you *truly* have unconditional permission to eat? Reflect on a recent time you allowed yourself to eat a forbidden food, and describe the experience. Did you place any conditions on allowing yourself to eat the forbidden food?

_____

_____

This is a tough question for many people. As you read the example below, gently connect with the statements to see if they might be true for you.

Perhaps you offered yourself pseudo-permission, that is, you placed conditions on how much you could eat, such as *I can eat just one cookie, but only if my weight is okay.* Or perhaps you made a deal to compensate for eating a forbidden food: *I can eat this slice of pie if I run five miles or if I eat less at the next meal.* This compensatory deal making places a condition on your eating in order to make it acceptable.

Or perhaps you found yourself in the whatever or what-the-hell style of eating. In this situation, you are behaviorally eating the forbidden food, but it is not unconditional permission to eat it. Rather, it reflects reactive eating—*I'll just eat it. I have to get it out of my system*—where ultimately, the intention is to get back in control, with tightened rules around the eating.

3. *I won't eat healthfully.* Eating healthy feels good. But when you believe that your opportunity to eat a forbidden food is now or never, the priority for health in that moment is fleeting, and it makes it more likely that you will eat in the absence of hunger. By making peace with a forbidden food, you will no longer overeat it or have anxiety about eating it. Because you have given yourself permission to eat a cookie, you will not be fraught with guilt. Consequently, you actually *taste* the cookie for the first time, and you might discover that it has little taste (very pretty, but no flavor) and decide not to eat it, or you might find that it is absolutely delicious and that it only takes one or two bites to satisfy you. But note: while you are still becoming familiar with Intuitive Eating and gaining confidence in your abilities, keep in mind that if you focus on nutritious eating too soon, you will likely embrace nutrition as another set of dieting rules. For the moment, put healthy eating on the back burner. We will concentrate on that later, after you've become an Intuitive Eater.

Reflect on how pursuing a healthy relationship with food could ultimately improve your health (even if it means allowing yourself to eat a restricted food).

_____

_____

4. *I am addicted to food.* Dieting is the gateway that makes forbidden foods even more enticing and difficult to stop eating. Food restrictions and hunger heighten the rewarding value of food, but that is not addiction, rather it's a compensatory reaction to deprivation—a rebound effect—and a biological response for survival. (See the sidebar later in this chapter, "What If You Believe You Are Addicted to Food?") Are there foods that you are uncomfortable eating, things that perhaps feel somewhat threatening, yet they seem to have an I-can't-stop-eating-them quality for you? List those foods here and consider beginning to make peace with those foods first.

    _____

    _____

5. *I don't trust myself around food.* Keep in mind that dieting undermines self-trust and connection with your body. It is dieting that has failed you and has perpetuated the feast-famine mentality. Trust takes time to cultivate, but it will grow every time you honor your hunger and take care of your basic needs. Your body has survived a nutritional trauma, and your cells need to know that they will be fed and taken care of, which will take repetition and consistency.

    Has there ever been a time in your life where eating was not an issue? Reflect on your eating behavior before you started dieting.

    _____

    _____

    On the other hand, if you were put on a diet at a very early age, with well-meaning parents monitoring every bit of food you put into your mouth, you may have internalized a powerful message that you cannot be trusted with food. In that situation, it would be understandable that you feel you cannot trust yourself around eating. You might truly be learning to eat and respond to your inner body signals for the first time in your life. If this is the case for you, what reassuring or compassionate statement can you tell yourself?

    _____

    _____

6. *My friends or family will criticize my food choices.* No single person could possibly know your thoughts, feelings, experiences, hunger, and fullness level, let alone what foods will satisfy you. Only you do. The process of becoming an Intuitive Eater is an inward journey, a solo endeavor, and even well-meaning comments and criticism from other people do not serve this connection. They do not need to understand the process, but it's important that they respect your journey. It may be helpful to set a boundary or ask for support from friends

and family. Describe what you could say to concerned family and friends if they comment on your food choices.

_____

_____

7. *I need to lose weight first.* This thought reflects the diet mentality. Remember that focusing on weight loss and dieting is at the root of the problem. Intuitive Eating is about healing your relationship with food, mind, and body, which may or may not result in weight loss. Focusing on weight loss will only prolong the problem, not help it. Describe what you could say to yourself to keep the focus on becoming an Intuitive Eater.

_____

_____

What If You Believe You Are Addicted to Food?

Can you really be addicted to food? That question is similar to asking if can you be addicted to breathing. Both eating and breathing are vital for life. Yet there is a prevalent belief that food addiction is a viable problem. The real problem is that the concept of food addiction is, at best, controversial, and it may hinder progress in identifying preventable causes of over-eating, such as dieting (Long, Blundell, and Finlayson 2015). There are many reasons other than addiction why food can seem irresistible and compelling to eat.

Food Is Supposed To Be Rewarding. Food is necessary for our survival. That's why, if you have been dieting or fasting for a medical procedure, you will likely have more thoughts and cravings for food. Fasting triggers the brain to ramp up dopamine, the feel-good neurohormone. A recent brain-imaging study on dieting teens showed that acute and prolonged caloric deprivation increases the reward value of food, particularly of calorie-rich, palatable foods. (Stice, Burger, and Yokum 2013).

Fasting Creates "Sugar-Addicted" Rats. A seminal study from Princeton University ignited interest in the concept of food addiction. Researchers induced rats to exhibit binge eating on sugar by depriving them of food for twelve hours, followed by a twelve-hour period with access to sugar and rat chow. That design is a very important detail that seldom gets reported. The *only* way the researchers were able to get this "addiction" effect was by starving the rats for twelve hours. Another group of rats were subject to the identical diet condition (chow and sugar), but they had no fasting period and had full access to their rat chow. These non-fasted rats did not binge on sugar (Carr 2011). The headlines on this study should have been "Food Restriction Causes Sugar-Binge."

Just Because Someone Uses the Term "Food Addiction," That Does Not Mean It Is a Fact. For example, consider the Yale Food Addiction Questionnaire (YFAS). Certainly an assessment tool from an esteemed university is proof that food addiction exists, yes? No. Long, Blundell, and Finlayson (2015) criticized it as being a circular argument—a logical fallacy—which goes like this:

Q: Why is this person a food addict?

A: Because of a high score on the YFAS.

Q: Why does this person score high on the YFAS?

A: Because he or she is a food addict.

When you take a closer look at the YFAS, the questions could actually reflect the consequences of food restriction and dieting! When the questionnaire was created and validated, the researchers did not control for dieting, which is a huge confounder (Gearhardt, Corbin, and Brownell 2009). In fact, a great majority of studies on food addiction do not control for dieting history.

Learned Conditioning, Not Addiction. Eating popcorn at the movies or peanuts at a baseball game are common examples of learned conditioning. Dr. Pavlov is famous for getting his dogs to salivate by simply ringing a bell. He achieved this by giving the dogs a treat every time he rang the bell. After repeated exposure, just hearing the bell was enough to get the dogs drooling. But there was an important follow-up to that study, which is not as well known. Pavlov deconditioned the dogs by ringing the bell but now not giving the dogs treats. Repeatedly. Consequently, the dogs uncoupled the sound of the bell with receiving treats. No more anticipatory salivation.

Lastly, when compulsive eaters eat forbidden foods as part of their treatment, their binge eating decreased markedly (Kristeller and Wolever 2011). Food addiction theory would predict otherwise.

ARE YOU READY TO MAKE PEACE WITH FOOD?

The purpose of the following questions is to help you assess your readiness to try new food experiences and challenges. Remember, this is not a pass or fail assessment. Rather, it serves to help you get a sense of your own readiness to venture out into new food experiences.

Yes	No	
		1. I have an environment in which I am able to eat unrushed and without distraction.
		2. I am able to identify key vulnerability points—such as being too hungry, too stressed out, too tired, and so forth.
		3. I am able to clearly identify my biological cues of hunger, ranging from ravenously empty to pleasant and gentle hunger.
		4. I can clearly identify my biological cues of fullness, ranging from gentle fullness to painfully stuffed.
		5. I can distinguish between the uncomfortable sensations of guilt versus the uncomfortable sensation of feeling too full.
		6. I am able to cope with my feelings without turning to food.
		7. I can distinguish between being hungry enough for a meal or just needing a snack.
		8. I am able to experience pleasurable satisfaction from eating a meal.
		9. I am able to tolerate the uncomfortable feeling of being too full from eating, without compensating by skipping a meal or exercising more.
		10. My food choices are not affected by the opinions of others.

REFLECTION: YOUR READINESS TO MAKE PEACE WITH FOOD

If you answered yes to most of the above questions, it indicates that you are ready to proceed with the peace process. Keep in mind that you still might not feel ready, even if you answered yes. That's okay. Some of these statements reflect Intuitive Eating principles that will be addressed in later chapters. It's understandable that you might not feel ready at this point. If you have not yet read *Intuitive Eating* (Tribole and Resch 2012), it would help you to understand the process and be more fully ready to tackle this issue. You might also find it helpful to read the rest of this workbook to learn how the practices are interconnected.

If you answered no to most of the questions—or if you just don't feel ready to proceed—it's important to progress at a pace that is comfortable to you. For example, if you are an emotional eater, you might want to focus on that issue first (see chapter 7, Cope with Your Feelings Without Using Food). Or if you are having difficulty with self-care (see chapter 2), you may need more time to have that foundation clearly established. Please be assured that with a little more practice, you will gain the necessary skills.

Keep in mind that you are not required to complete or master the principles of Intuitive Eating in any particular order. You need to do what is right for you and your situation. Some readers might find some principles easier than others, and some might need to work more slowly and carefully through some chapters. If, after you have finished this book, you still feel you need assistance, know that there are health care professionals who specialize in Intuitive Eating (see the directory of certified Intuitive Eating counselors in the list of resources at the end of this book).

SYSTEMATIC HABITUATION: MAKE PEACE WITH FOOD

The goal of unconditional permission to eat is not to burn out on the food, so that you'll never want to eat it again (that is actually a form of deprivation). Rather, the objective is to remove the excitement of the forbidden-fruit syndrome through systematic habituation. Making peace with food is actually a form of exposure therapy, which involves systematically confronting a fear (in this case, food) so that erroneous beliefs about its danger are repudiated (Harned et al. 2014).

There are many ways to make peace with food. But it goes more smoothly if we harness what we have learned from habituation research. For example, we know that novelty, variety, and distraction delay the habituation process. So it is helpful to eat without distraction and to choose the same food and same flavor before moving on to another food. For example, if you wanted to make peace with ice cream, it's best to choose one flavor rather than buying a variety of flavors. Varying the flavor (or even the brand) extends the period of novelty—it's almost like starting anew with each flavor, even though it's the same kind of food.

You will likely need to repeat this process several times—with the same food, as well as with different forbidden foods. This is not a race, and it's important to proceed at a pace that is comfortable for you. Also, rest assured that you will not need to eat your way down the alphabet, testing out every single forbidden food. Rather, after many experiences of eating a few different forbidden foods, there will be a shift—you truly know that you can eat whatever food you like. No further proof or experimentation will be needed at that point. This will depend on the chronicity of your dieting experiences, which is different for everyone, but everyone can get there. It's important to have patience and compassion for yourself in this process.

Getting Ready: Prepare to Make the Best of Your Experience

Complete the following questionnaire in order to help you to get ready to make peace with food in a systematic manner.

Preparation

Choose a time when you are not likely to be too hungry (such as an hour after a meal):

_____

Choose a specific food (consider the brand and flavor):

_____

Decide where you will eat the food:

☐ Home ☐ Out ☐ Kitchen ☐ Dining room ☐ Other _____

What do you need in order to feel safe eating a forbidden food? Perhaps a low-stress day in a calm environment? Perhaps support from your roommate, family, or friends?

_____

Checking In During the Process

It's important to stay connected with your experiences during the peace process. Here are some things to think about.

Before: Take note of what you feel before you begin your eating experience? (Excitement? Dread? Worry? Curiosity?)

_____

_____

During: How is the taste? Texture? Is this taste and texture meeting your expectations?

_____

_____

After: Any surprises? Overall, did the experience of eating this food meet your expectations? Would you do anything differently?

_____

_____

Milestones Chart

The purpose of this chart is to help you track your progress of making peace with food at a glance. Use this chart to record any milestone in which you gave yourself permission to eat a feared food and felt the experience was a success. Record the date and the challenge food, and describe your experience.

Date	Food	Experience
Example	Cookies	*Gave myself permission to eat cookies. I ate only two bites, because the taste was disappointing. Surprised how effortless this was.*
Example	Dessert	*Ate dinner at a restaurant that is famous for its cheesecake. I gave myself permission to eat dessert. The cheesecake was incredibly delicious. I stopped after four bites, because I was full. I felt sad and pulled to eat more, but then I told myself that I can eat it with my lunch tomorrow, and I stopped.*
Example	Sandwich	*I gave myself permission to eat bread (big fear food) by eating a sandwich at lunch, rather than a big salad. I was scared, but so surprised how it sustained me until dinner, with no afternoon craving for something sweet.*

A Couple Final Notes

Entitlement Eating (You Can't Tell Me What to Eat)

This type of eating is driven by rebellion, with little attunement to hunger and fullness. While you might argue and rationalize it—*I can eat it because I want to*—it can be a form of reactive, disconnected eating. There tends to be a particular energy associated with this type of eating—it's intense and rebellious. But this type of eating is not usually very satisfying, because it's not really about the taste or attunement; rather, it's about making a statement. It is a trap and distorts the premise of Intuitive Eating. Just remember you have nothing to prove—to yourself or to others.

What About Allergies and Medical Conditions

The types of forbidden foods that are the most problematic for rebound eating are those that are self-imposed for weight loss. Sometimes, of course, there are medical conditions that would cause some foods to be off-limits—such as a life-threatening allergy to peanuts, or celiac disease, which is an autoimmune disorder that can only be treated by eating a gluten-free diet. Under these conditions, it is likely that you may feel a level of deprivation, as you are no longer free to eat certain foods without an adverse physical reaction. Remember, Intuitive Eating is about listening to all of the messages your body gives you and striving to feel good in your body as a result of your food choices. As you become an intuitive eater, your body will come to respond to foods that make it feel good, and so if you are in tune with your body, you will want those forbidden foods less. If you continue to have an emotional reaction, it is important to discuss this with your therapist and/or nutritionist. If you have less access to food as a result of financial limits, it is important to discuss your feelings, as well.

You may also feel some level of deprivation if you eliminate some foods for ethical or moral reasons. It is likely, however, that your philosophical convictions will take precedence over the deprivation.

If you are unsure about your medical condition and the foods you eat, please be sure to consult with your health care team.

Wrap-Up

In this chapter, you learned how to make peace with food and why it is a critical component of Intuitive Eating. Psychological deprivation of food can trigger a rebound effect, causing you to overeat forbidden foods. When this type of deprivation is combined with the dieting mentality and biological hunger, once you take the first bite of the verboten food, it can seem impossible to stop eating. Legalizing your food choices through the process of habitation removes the thrill and urgency of eating the forbidden fruit. It calms your fears that you'll never stop eating it. Ultimately, it's a process of placing value on your emotional health and removing the morality from eating while increasing the flexibility of your food choices.

In the next chapter, you will learn how powerful your thoughts are when it comes to feelings and ultimately how your thinking affects your eating behavior.

CHAPTER 4

Principle Four
Challenge the Food Police

The food police monitor the unreasonable rules that dieting has created. The police station is housed deep in your psyche, and its loudspeaker shouts negative barbs, hopeless phrases, and guilt-provoking indictments. Chasing the food police away is a critical step in returning to Intuitive Eating.

In this chapter, you will learn how to silence the instigator of the war with food, which are your thoughts that form the voice of what we call the food police. These thoughts and food rules do not just appear in your mind out of nowhere. They become internalized as a result of a variety of factors.

We are all born into this world innocent, filled with instinct and emotions and the capacity to eventually form thoughts. Even in the womb, the child learns about the world. Smells, voices, and sensations can be experienced, but the formulation of a belief system about the world begins once the child is influenced by the environment outside the womb. Beliefs about people, politics, religion, culture, education, and so forth, to which a child is exposed while growing up, are the building blocks of the child's early formation of his or her own beliefs. In the realm of eating, this child lives in a nation—and, perhaps, a home—riddled with guilt about eating. Foods are often described in moralistic terms: decadent, sinful, tempting, or bad. This way of viewing food has become a false religion. Dieting has become the absolving ritual for removing the guilt of eating pleasurable foods.

The key defense for challenging the food police is to first develop nonjudgmental awareness of your thoughts and then cultivate retorts to the food police's judgments and demands. Learning to speak up is essential to your self-esteem. The exercises in this chapter will provide ways to address and reframe those negative thoughts, so that the food police retreat and, ultimately, vanish.

Examine Your Beliefs

We have introjected the societal food police—the collective cultural voice—which becomes our inner food police. We know where to find it—it actually doesn't have a very clever hiding place. It's in the forefront of your mind and may sometimes feel as if it's sitting on your shoulder, like Jiminy Cricket, whose favorite phrase was "let your conscience be your guide."

You may have spent your life cowering before the voices from a critical parent, teacher, or spouse, only to have those voices internalized and made into your own. Consequently, your mind becomes clouded with self-doubt and negative thinking.

The solution is to examine your beliefs—their origin and impact on you—as these beliefs are the springboard for the thoughts of the food police. You will learn how these thoughts affect your feelings and, ultimately, behavior.

Evaluate Your Belief System About Food and Your Body

Review this list of prevalent distorted beliefs. Place a check by the statements that fall within your belief system.

☐ Protein is the best food group.

☐ Fats in food make the food fattening and will make me fat.

☐ Carbohydrates are unnecessary to eat during the day.

☐ People should never eat foods with white flour or sugar.

☐ Everyone knows that gluten is bad for you.

☐ People have to be skinny in order to find a perfect partner, job, acting role, and so forth.

☐ Diets are the most efficient way to lose weight.

☐ Eating after six at night will cause me to gain weight.

List any other beliefs you have about food and your body:

_____

_____

_____

_____

Examine the Origin of Your Beliefs

Beliefs are cultivated and influenced by many factors. For example, many people have a family history of living with a focus on weight and body size. A mother might comment on how her child looks and how the child's clothing fits. A parent may use the scale daily and talk about dieting. A grandparent might make admonitions about how much food her grandchild is eating. There might be magazines in the home full of celebrity photographs that have been digitally altered to make their bodies look perfect.

Reflect upon the origin of your beliefs about your body or eating:

_____

_____

_____

_____

_____

Beliefs Affect Thoughts

Your thoughts are formulated from the set of beliefs you hold about how the world around you works. The thoughts and rules spoken by the food police are usually *cognitive distortions*—very strong statements that are based on false beliefs. If not challenged, these negative thoughts can affect many of your behaviors, especially your eating.

Examine Your Thoughts

Here are some examples of cognitive distortions. Read each one, and reflect on whether you've ever had a similar thought:

- *I should never eat carbohydrates during the day, even if I crave them.*

- *It would be okay to eat fruits and vegetables for carbs—that's good. But it's bad to eat bread or pasta.*

- *I will never find the perfect partner unless I lose weight and become skinny.*

- *Since I can't stay on a diet, I must be a loser!*

- *Maybe there's a diet out there that will end up working for me.*

Have you had other exaggerated thoughts? Write down any that come to mind.

_____

_____

_____

_____

Challenge Your Food Police Thoughts

There are two keys ways to work with food police thoughts. The first method, cognitive behavioral therapy (CBT), is the focus of this section.

CBT involves evaluating your thoughts and reframing them if they are faulty, which ultimately affects your behavior. The process begins with your observing your thoughts and questioning whether a thought is reasonable. Is there any scientific evidence to support your thought? Or does it sound unjustifiable, unreasonable, and faulty? Once you have identified an unreasonable or illogical thought, challenge it by replacing it with a logical thought.

Reflecting on your actual past experiences will help you evaluate whether your present thought has any truth or accuracy and whether it has actually resulted in any benefit to you. Here are some examples of a distorted thought, followed by a reframing of that thought, based on your past experience:

Unreasonable thought—a cognitive distortion:

I should never eat carbohydrates during the day, even if I crave them.

Questions to ask:

Should I really never eat carbohydrates?

Aren't there times of the day when I do, in fact, eat a lot of carbs?

How do I feel when I don't eat any carbohydrates during the day?

Thought reframed, based on past experiences:

My past experience demonstrates that when I haven't eaten carbohydrates during the day, I end up having little energy and often binge on carbs at night.

Reflection upon the result of acting on your reframed thought:

Since I've added carbs to my meals throughout the day, I've stopped binging on cookies and chips at night, and I feel so much better all day.

Unreasonable thought—a cognitive distortion:

It would be okay to eat fruits and vegetables—that's good. But it's bad to eat bread or pasta.

Questions to ask:

Has eating pasta actually ever harmed me?

How do I feel when I only eat fruits and vegetables as my carbs?

Thought reframed, based on past experiences:

When I have only eaten fruits and vegetables to get my carbohydrates, I'm not able to sustain my energy throughout the day.

Reflection:

Now that I've included cereal and sandwiches in my meals, I can think more clearly and stay alert throughout the day. Eating only fruits and vegetables didn't work for me!

Your Turn: Practice Reframing Thoughts with Actual Experience

Describe a common distorted thought about your eating. Ask some questions related to this thought, reframe it with your actual experience, and reflect upon it:

Distorted thought:

_____

_____

Questions to ask:

_____

_____

Thought reframed based on your actual experience:

_____

_____

Reflection:

_____

_____

Make Statements Based on Facts

A second way you can challenge cognitive distortions or myths is by reframing them with facts. Here is an example:

Distortion: *I will never find the perfect partner unless I lose weight and become skinny.*

Reframed: *I have several friends who are in happy relationships who are not skinny.*

Your Turn: Practice Reframing Your Distorted Thoughts with Facts

What are some faulty thoughts you carry? Reframe them with fact-based thoughts:

Distorted thought:

_____

_____

Reframed statement based on facts:

_____

_____

Distorted thought:

_____

_____

Reframed statement based on facts:

_____

_____

Approach Your Thoughts with Curious Awareness

The second way to work with food police thoughts is a simple process of just observing your thoughts, without allowing them to occupy your mind and without passing any judgment on them. Simply observe them. This is a form of mindfulness called *curious awareness*. Our minds habitually take hold of a thought and build a narrative or story around it, which can create unnecessary suffering. A robust body of research shows that using curious awareness, through mindfulness-based meditation, can be incredibly beneficial to your mental health (Grecucci et al. 2015). Simply observe your thoughts, without attaching to them or adding to the story line.

Your Turn: Practice Approaching Your Thoughts with Curious Awareness

Notice when you're expanding your thoughts with a story you've created. Write an example of a root thought. Reflect on how adding a judgmental thought or a narrative story line makes you feel:

_____

_____

_____

_____

When the same (or a similar) root thought arises, try to observe it without adding a narrative or judgment. There are many ways to practice doing this:

- Place your awareness on the present moment, rather than the thought. Pay attention to one of your senses, such as sight, touch, or sound.

- Simply label the thought as "thinking" or "mere thoughts, not facts."

- Consider learning and developing a regular meditation practice.

Pick one of these methods to practice and note how it feels:

_____

_____

_____

_____

You have practiced ways in which you can challenge your food police thoughts, as well as the benefits of curious awareness. Depending on the individual situation at hand, one method may be more useful than another. By reframing your thoughts based on past eating experiences and by making statements based on facts, you can challenge an unreasonable thought. Additionally, you can reduce any suffering caused by a distorted thought by approaching it with neutral awareness, without attaching to it or creating a story around it.

How Thoughts Affect Feelings

Just as beliefs inform your thoughts, your thoughts can have a powerful impact on your feelings. Let's say that you realize that you're feeling anxious. If you explore the thought that preceded that feeling, it might be, *I ate too much today*. By evaluating and challenging that thought, the ensuing feeling is likely to be more neutral or even positive.

Pay Attention to Your Feelings

Here is a list of feelings that are often connected with eating and your body:

- anxiety

- sadness

- fear

- disappointment

- remorse

- envy

- anger

- shame

Refer back to the negative thoughts you noted in the Examine Your Thoughts exercise earlier in this chapter. Reflect on one of these thoughts and notice if it creates any of the above feelings.

_____

_____

_____

Reframe Your Negative, Judgmental Thoughts

The exercise below will help you recognize the impact of thoughts on your feelings. By reframing the thoughts, you can change your feelings.

First, describe how you feel after reading these negative statements:

- *I am a loser—I can never stay on a diet!*

- *I'm always overeating!*

- *I told myself not to eat carbs, and I just ate a whole box of cookies!*

_____

_____

_____

Next, notice and describe how you feel when these negative thoughts are reframed into positive statements:

- *The system of dieting is a set-up for failure, and I have rejected it! I'm not a loser!*

- *When I'm mindful, I often notice my hunger and fullness, because I have the innate ability to detect both.*

- *With full permission to choose to eat whatever food I desire, I eat reasonable amounts of cookies.*

_____

_____

Now, reexamine your feelings. Compare and contrast your feelings, before and after expressing a positive statement:

_____

_____

_____

You have learned the powerful impact that challenging a negative thought can have on your overall well-being. The more you transform negative thoughts into positive thoughts, the less flooded you'll be with negative feelings.

How Feelings Affect Behavior

You have experienced the impact that your belief system can have on your thoughts and how your thoughts can affect your feelings. Now, it's time to understand how feelings (either positive or negative) can influence your behavior.

Reflect on Past Overeating Experiences

Reflect on a recent experience when you overate and ended up feeling uncomfortable. What did you eat, and where were you?

_____

_____

_____

Recollect what feelings you were having just before you began to overeat. Were they negative, positive, or indifferent?

_____

_____

_____

How did those feelings impact your overeating behavior?

_____

_____

If you had negative feelings, they were likely triggered by negative thoughts, and those feelings might have impacted your behavior. Beliefs can initiate a cascade of negativity. Examining these beliefs can be your first step to changing the course of your actions in the future. Don't forget: beliefs create thoughts, which affect feelings and then behavior. Practicing this exercise will empower you and give you a sense of agency in your ability to shift your eating behaviors into new ones that will be positive and enjoyable.

Spiral of Healing—The Way Out of Judgmental Self-Talk

Come From a Place of Curiosity, Not Judgment

Intuitive Eating involves a neutral, appreciative way of thinking. It's filled with positive thoughts and gratitude. It's based on the process of making change at one's own pace. People who live with the diet mentality often have black-and-white thinking and see life in a linear way. They approach projects with the goal of going from A to Z in a straight line, rather than flowing with the ups and downs that come with any realistic goal in life. In the diet mentality, there is no room for deviation along the path. But life doesn't work that way, and when the inevitable deviation occurs, the dieter's rigid thinking leads to a sense of bewilderment and negative self-talk for not being able to stay on course. Negative beliefs and thinking impact your mental health.

Intuitive Eating gives you a more compassionate way of looking at your journey toward a healthy relationship with food. Imagine Intuitive Eating as a spiral of healing (see figure 4.1). The momentum is upward and onward, but it doesn't flow in a straight line. It circles around the loops of the spiral as it moves upward. Those little loops represent moments of returning to past behaviors. These moments allow for reflection—time to examine beliefs and thoughts, self-care, and negative self-talk. All of these loops may have precipitated what some would label a setback, but which burgeoning Intuitive Eaters come to see as learning experiences. Make your motto "Come from a place of curiosity, not judgment!"

Spiral of Healing

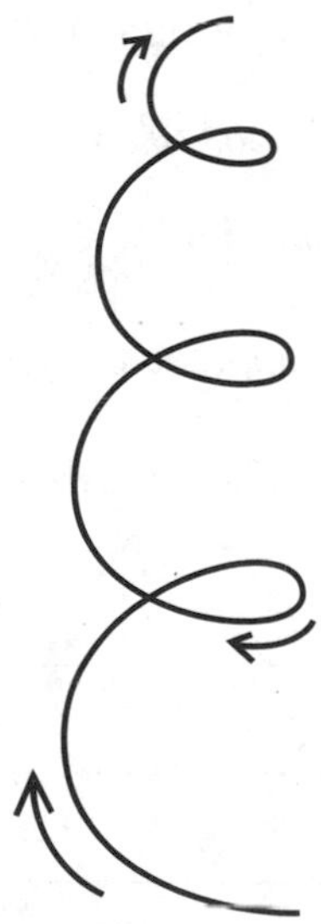

Figure 4.1.   The Spiral of Healing.
© 2017 Elyse Resch / New Harbinger Publications.

Transforming Negative Self-Talk into Positive Self-Talk and Gratitude

Consider the ways in which you engage in negative self-talk. For example, *I'm worthless, because I don't meet my exercise goals.* Provide an example of your own:

_____

_____

_____

CREATE POSITIVE SELF-TALK AND GRATITUDE

Describe how you could change the negative self-talk you listed above into positive self-talk, using the concepts of the spiral of healing. Remember to come from a place of curiosity, not judgment. For the example above, you might say, *I'm so proud of myself for bringing movement into my life. I'm not doing it consistently, but I'm working on it. I'm amazing!*

_____

_____

_____

Expressing gratitude is another way of moving from negativity to positivity.

- *I am fortunate to be able to buy fresh food whenever I need to fill my refrigerator.*

- *I am grateful for the strong body I have, which gets me through life.*

- *I feel lucky to have a more nurturing approach to food.*

Make your own gratitude list. How does seeing the world through the lens of gratitude impact you and your life?

_____

_____

_____

_____

_____

Frame Your Goals and Behaviors with "For the Most Part" Thinking

The most common trap in which clients get stuck is perfectionistic thinking. This premise must be reframed in order to remove negative self-talk. Whenever you attempt to do something *every day* or *always*, your goal is perfection. Keep in mind Salvador Dali's adage: "Have no fear of perfection—you'll never reach it." Here are some examples of perfectionistic thinking:

- *I'm going to start exercising and go for a run every day next week.*

- *I won't ever put anything in my mouth unless I feel that distinct hunger signal.*

- *I will always stop when I'm full and never overeat.*

Realistically, how long do you think you will be able to keep up these types of commitments? And what happens when your child is eating a cookie and wants to share it with you, or when your partner says, "Let's go out to lunch now," but you're barely hungry? The problem with these goals is that the moment you don't reach your perfectionist standard, you feel as if you've blown it. You might even feel shame that you can't be true to your word. With this disappointment in yourself and the accompanying shame, you're likely to give up on your goal entirely.

One way of reframing your thinking is by adopting the phrase "for the most part." When you set your goals, include a bit of flexibility: *I'm going to exercise as often as it feels good, and when I'm too tired or don't have time, I'll rest.* In other words, remember your commitment to consistent movement is going to be "for the most part."

If you set out the intention that you'll eat primarily when you're hungry, acknowledge that there might be circumstances that warrant eating something even if you're not quite there. For the most part, you're eating for hunger, but you're also going to decide to eat just for pleasure or convenience now and then.

Practicing the "For the Most Part" Frame of Mind

Reframe the following perfectionist goals into intentions of "for the most part." Write a more reasonable intention, something that will have the likelihood of being successful. For example:

Perfectionist goal: *I am going to always eat intuitively!*

For the most part intention: *I will regularly stay mindful while eating and hope that, for the most part, I will be an Intuitive Eater.*

Now, you try making this shift for the following statements:

I'm going to eat only organic food.

_____

_____

_____

I'm going to tell myself that I look beautiful every single day.

_____

_____

_____

_____

I'm going to get up at six every morning to exercise.

_____

_____

_____

_____

Create your own intention using "for the most part" thinking.

_____

_____

_____

_____

Keep this pattern of thinking in mind in whatever you are doing. In fact, make a list of your "for the most part" intentions and post it where you'll see it easily. It will eliminate perfectionist thinking—for the most part!

Food Rules

As a result of diet thinking, you may have created many food rules, which are based on old beliefs. They may have accumulated over your lifetime. Many people say that a powerful source of these beliefs and rules was their upbringing or the dynamics of their family when they were children. In this section, you will explore these food rules, which are spoken by the food police, and evaluate how these rules can affect you.

Examine Your Food Rules

No one starts out in life with "Ten Commandments of Eating," engraved in stone, that must be obeyed. Belief systems and rules of eating evolve subtly. The questionnaire below will put you in touch with your food rules. Read the checklist, check yes or no, and fill in the blank spaces with any of your own food rules.

What Are Your Food Rules?

Yes	No	
		1. Do you count anything (calories, fat, carbs, protein, points, and so forth)?
		2. Do calories determine how much you eat?
		3. Do you feel you have to eat perfectly to be a healthy eater?
		4. Do you have any rules about what time of day is okay to eat?
		5. Do you have any rules about snacking?
		6. Are there any foods that you try to avoid?
		7. Do you have any rules about knowing the nutrition content of a meal or food?
		8. Do you eat differently if there are other people present?
		9. Do you compare what you eat to what other people are eating?
		10. Do you have any rules around beverages?
		11. Do you have any rules around exercise and eating?
		12. Do you believe that carbs should be limited?
		13. Do you think that sweets should be avoided?
		14. Do you weigh or measure your food?
		15. Do you have a list of "safe" foods to eat?
		16.
		17.

On the lines below, or in a separate notebook, write out the questions that you marked with a yes, and explore your answers, explaining how you fulfill that rule in your life. For the moment, don't ask yourself why you do this or look into ways of eliminating or changing this rule.

Example: Question 3. Do you feel you have to eat perfectly to be a healthy eater? *Yes. I eat perfectly by eating very few carbs and very low fat, and I eat no gluten.*

_____

_____

_____

_____

Challenge Your Food Rules

Review your answers, and see if you can reframe your food rules with answers that are flexible and not absolute. Notice when your thoughts have been rigid or perfectionist. For some questions, see if you can add "for the most part" to your answers. For example, *I know that I can trust my body to give me the signals that will lead to balanced, healthy eating—for the most part.* For others, you will find that the healthiest intention you can set is to challenge the food rule entirely. For example, you may have answered yes to *Do you think that sweets should be avoided?* In this case, reframing that rule with Intuitive Eating thinking would be, *I've made peace with all foods, and I can eat sweets whenever I like—no foods need to be avoided.*

_____

_____

_____

_____

Your Family's Food Rules

Your family's beliefs have a powerful influence on forming your belief system. Even if their intentions are entirely positive, many parents raise their kids with rules about what's okay and not okay to eat. It's important to get a sense of these rules from your childhood, their degree of rigidity, and how they might still be affecting you. (Note: if you are a child or a teen, and thus are exploring the nutrition rules that you see around you, remember that your parents were likely well meaning when creating them.) As you read the checklist below in the questionnaire, take some time to reflect on each question before you answer yes or no.

What Were Your Family's Rules and Expectations?

Yes	No	Types of Questions to Ask
		1. Did your parents have rigid rules for eating family meals?
		2. Were you expected to clean your plate?
		3. Were there any rules about snacking?
		4. Were there any rules about eating sweets or desserts?
		5. Were there any forbidden foods? For example, were you not allowed to eat sweets or fast food?
		6. Did you ever sneak food when your parents weren't around?
		7. Did you feel excited at friends' parties because of the opportunity to eat goodies when your parents weren't around?
		8. Was there a lot of pressure about your weight?
		9. Did your mom and dad seem to have different food rules for you as opposed to rules for themselves?
		10. Did you ever get mixed messages from your parents? For example, did they warn you not to eat too much—saying that you would gain weight—yet they insisted on your finishing your plate, even if you were not hungry?
		11. Did your parents have any rules about exercise?
		12. Did one or both of your parents diet frequently?
		13. Did one or both of your parents criticize their own body frequently?
		14. Did your parents monitor your weight?
		15. Did your parents ever put you on a diet?

Review Your Responses to Your Family's Food Rules

On the lines below, or in a notebook, write down questions to which you answered yes, and describe how the rule was applied in your house and the consequences of these rules.

Example: Question 2. Were you expected to clean your plate? *Yes, my parents wouldn't let us kids leave the dinner table until we finished every bite. If we didn't finish, we had to sit there—sometimes for hours—before we could go. Sometimes we'd try to feed some of our food to the dog or hide it in our napkins, but if we were found out, we were punished!*

_____

_____

_____

_____

Distinguish Your Own Beliefs from Your Family's Rules

Look at each of your answers above, and for each answer, write down how you feel about these family rules and expectations. A possible statement reflecting your current thinking might look something like this: *I finish eating when my body tells me I'm full. I would only continue eating until my plate was empty, if I were still hungry.*

_____

_____

_____

_____

Comments from Others

Have family members, friends, or acquaintances made comments about your weight, shape, or what or how much you're eating? If the person making this comment acts like a critical parent, it is likely that you will feel like a rebellious child, and your behavior may reflect these feelings.

Reflect on the Impact of Comments from Others

A critical comment that could have a powerful effect might be something like: "That outfit is not very flattering on you" or "Do you really need that entire steak?" Would you feel an instinct to rebel against this comment? Rebellious energy, if not addressed, can create a backlash, which often takes the form of overeating. And would you also respond in other ways, feeling hurt, angry, resentful, or scared in response to the comment?

_____

_____

How do you normally respond to a person who makes a comment like one of these?

_____

_____

_____

Although you can't control others, you can speak up and assert that these types of statements hurt you or make you angry. Even if the person making the comment defends it by saying, "I'm only worried about your health," the critical comment is hurtful and is crossing into your personal space. If you are not heard, and the person continues to be inappropriately critical or mean, you don't have to stay and take it. In some instances, you'll find that you can set boundaries, and the person might actually honor them. In either case, you can feel empowered by taking an assertive action, rather than acting out rebelliously.

EXPLORE COMMENTS YOU HAVE RECEIVED FROM OTHERS

Write down a specific comment you have received from a parent, friend, partner, or someone else.

_____

_____

_____

How did you feel when you heard that comment?

_____

_____

_____

What action did you take? What did you say or do?

_____

_____

_____

Was there any other action you wish you had taken? If so, what would that be?

_____

_____

_____

Repeat the steps in this exercise as often as you need. As a result, you will strengthen your armor in reacting to inappropriate comments. You will learn how to speak up, set boundaries, and truly take care of yourself.

Change Your Critical and Rebellious Self-Talk

You often cannot control how others speak to you, even if you confront them about their criticism, but you can change how you speak to yourself. If you speak to yourself in a critical way, it is likely that you will respond with a rebellious voice, just as you would if someone else spoke to you in this way.

Think about how you tend to speak to yourself and how you respond to that self-talk. Imagine that you thought to yourself, *You had a fattening hamburger for lunch, so you better not eat too much for dinner!* How would that self-talk make you feel?

_____

_____

_____

_____

Next, imagine that you responded to the above statement with the following retort: *Oh, yeah, I'll eat as much as I want for dinner—I might even eat another hamburger, and this time, I'll have fries with it!* Describe below how you feel when you imagine making that response. Do you feel like a rebellious child or teenager who is speaking in a defiant way?

_____

_____

_____

The following is a restatement of both inner voices. Pay attention to how you feel when you read it, and then, below, describe the feelings this statement invokes. *I am satisfied from that wonderful hamburger that I had at lunch, and I'm not feeling hungry right now. Dinnertime is coming up soon, and at that point I'll figure out what I feel like eating. If I'm hungry and feel like having a hamburger again, I just might do that. But I might just feel like eating a salad.*

_____

_____

_____

Regularly practicing this kind of restatement takes away the power of critical self-talk. You will find that as you speak to yourself more gently, you reduce your rebellious retorts.

Now think about the impact of this next example of self-talk. Imagine that you make this statement to yourself about your appearance: *You look so awful today. Your hair is stringy, your clothes aren't ironed, and you look fat!*

How did you feel as you read those words? Did you feel hurt, angry, resentful, or scared? What reaction would you normally have to that voice inside of you, which is speaking to you so critically? Might it be rebelliousness? If so, you are having an expected reaction.

_____

_____

_____

If you are using a critical voice toward yourself, practice replacing it with an objective, neutral voice. First, jot down a recurrent critical thought you have had about food, eating, or your body. Next, write how your neutral voice would replace that thought. For example, if you regularly tell yourself, *You shouldn't have eaten so much,* a kinder thought might be, *When I get distracted and eat more than my body needs, I feel uncomfortable. I'll work on being more mindful in order to feel better.*

_____

_____

_____

By noticing how you feel when you speak to yourself and when you respond to yourself or others, you will remove many of the barriers that have blocked you from connecting with the voice of your Intuitive Eater. It's the voice of your autonomous Intuitive Eater—who knows the truth of your thoughts and feelings—that will lead you to a healthy relationship with food and your body.

Inner Food Voices

We carry within us a number of different voices that direct and sometimes interfere with our intuitive signals. In this book, we have already discussed the voice of the food police, but there are other voices as well, and some are positive voices that can help us make informed decisions about our eating. We call all of these voices the *Inner Food Voices*. They are divided into two groups, the *Destructive Dieting Voices* and the *Powerful Ally Voices*.

The Destructive Dieting Voices can bring you down in a moment. You can, however, take these negative voices and transform them into Powerful Ally Voices by using some of the exercises you have been practicing to challenge your distorted thoughts.

The Destructive Dieting Voices have a detrimental effect on your relationship with food and your body:

- The *Food Police* decide whether you're being bad or good in relation to your food choices. It combines your dieting rules with your food rules.

- The *Nutrition Informant* aligns with the pervading cultural myths about which foods are healthy (not fattening) or unhealthy (fattening).

- The *Diet Rebel* makes rebellious comments that leave you feeling powerless in your ability to make autonomous decisions about your eating.

The *Powerful Ally Voices* can aid and comfort you in your relationship with food and your body:

- The *Food Anthropologist* is a neutral observer who makes comments without judgment.

- The *Nurturer* is the loving, kind voice that provides the most positive self-talk.

- The *Nutrition Ally* has a neutral voice that helps you make decisions about foods that will give you energy, health, and satiety, along with satisfaction.

- The *Intuitive Eater* is the voice that will come from your internal wisdom and will guide you to make the best choice for your body's needs.

Become Familiar with the Inner Food Voices

Here is a quiz to practice identifying the different food voices. Which voice is speaking in each of the following statements?

1. *If you eat that piece of cheese, you're going to get high cholesterol.*

2. *I'm going to eat all of these cookies, even though I'm not hungry and they're not really my favorite kind.*

3. *I can trust my body to tell me what to eat, when to eat, and how much to eat.*

4. *That food has a lot of garlic and onion in it, and I know that I get a stomachache every time I eat those foods.*

5. *I noticed that I was overly full all day yesterday.*

6. *Even though I ate past my fullness last night, it's all going to be okay.*

7. *I ate pizza last night, and I know I've gained five pounds from it!*

Answer key: 1. Nutrition Informant, 2. Diet Rebel, 3. Intuitive Eater, 4. Nutrition Ally, 5. Food Anthropologist, 6. Nurturer, 7. Food Police.

Observe Your Own Food Voices

Describe two examples of your self-talk about eating from recent days. After each statement, identify whether it came from a destructive voice or an ally voice.

Self-talk: _____

_____

_____

Destructive or ally voice? _____

Self-talk: _____

_____

_____

Destructive or ally voice? _____

By focusing on finding the destructive and ally voices we carry around, it helps us recognize them immediately when they pop up unannounced. We can then learn to replace a destructive voice with an ally voice.

Replace the Destructive Dieting Voices with the Powerful Ally Voices

Identify two of your common destructive statements. How would your corresponding ally voice respond?

Destructive statement: _____

_____

_____

Ally voice response: _____

_____

_____

Destructive statement:_____

_____

_____

Ally voice response: _____

_____

_____

Practice making these responses every time you hear a destructive voice in your head. By doing this exercise regularly, you'll find that the destructive voices appear less frequently, and, ultimately, you will hear only the ally voices.

Discover Your Innate Intuitive Eater Voice

You have just practiced reframing your destructive dieting voices by employing your powerful ally voices, which produce positive and encouraging self-talk. Ultimately, the goal is to uncover the voice of your innate Intuitive Eater and use it to guide you toward satisfying eating. Remember, you were born with all the wisdom you need to know how to eat. The voice of your Intuitive Eater will help you feel safe and confident about what to eat, how much to eat, and when to eat. For example, your Intuitive Eater will provide guiding and encouraging statements if you are planning to go out for a delicious dinner one night:

- *I'm going to a wonderful restaurant this evening, so I want to be sure to have an afternoon snack, so I won't walk into the restaurant feeling ravenous.*

- *When I get to the restaurant, I'll take some time to thoroughly look through the menu to find something which I hope will satisfy my taste buds and my body.*

- *When I feel comfortably full, I'll take some time to reflect on how delicious the food was and how great I'll feel if I stop eating at that point.*

- *I can take my leftovers home and enjoy them tomorrow. Or if they don't look good tomorrow, I can always just throw them out.*

- *I might feel sad when I realize that my body has had enough to eat but that my tongue still wants more, but I know that this sadness will pass quickly and that I can eat whatever I want when I get hungry again.*

Describe how your Intuitive Eater voice would respond in the following situations:

Situation: *I know that I would like some dessert after my meal.*

Intuitive Eater Voice Response: _____

_____

Situation: *I'm not feeling well this morning. What should I do about my plan to exercise today?*

Intuitive Eater Voice Response: _____

_____

Situation: *I have a fancy gala this coming Saturday night. How should I approach what I eat that night?*

Intuitive Eater Voice Response: _____

_____

Now, explore one of your real life situations:

Your Situation: _____

_____

Your Intuitive Eater Voice Response: _____

_____

Wrap-Up

Your war with food has been instigated by the voice of the food police. The exercises in this chapter are fundamental for learning how to challenge your negative thoughts, which, cumulatively, have formed the voice of your internal food police. By reframing these thoughts, you will finally silence the food police and make a lasting peace with food.

In the next chapter, you will see how the work you have done to reject the diet mentality, make peace with food, and challenge the food police will enable you to detect comfortable fullness, without the fear of future deprivation.

CHAPTER 5

Principle Five
Feel Your Fullness

Listen for the body signals that tell you that you are no longer hungry. Observe the signs that show that you're comfortably full. Pause in the middle of eating and ask yourself how the food tastes and what your current fullness level is.

It is difficult to identify fullness if you are eating while distracted, stuck in habitual patterns of cleaning your plate, or eating quickly without savoring your food. In the book *CrazyBusy* (2007), Edward M. Hallowell describes our modern predicament: people are incredibly busy and distracted, thanks to technology that's always on and a growing sense of urgency that we must be productive at all times. We always have to be doing something. Some people even view sitting down to simply enjoy a meal as a waste of time; they use their mealtimes to get other things done, even if it's just watching the news.

The activities in this chapter will help you to

- connect with your physical sensations from fullness;

- contemplate how you want to feel, physically, after eating a meal or snack;

- practice identifying the nuances of fullness;

- learn how to say no to people who pressure you to eat when you are either full or not yet hungry; and

- work on the clean-your-plate mentality.

Barriers to Experiencing Fullness

This section describes the many barriers that can make it difficult to hear your body's signal of fullness, from distracted eating to social pressure to eating past fullness. More importantly, you will practice ways to overcome the obstacles so that you can respond to your fullness signals in a timely manner.

Distracted Eating

Eating while engaged in another activity is much like distracted driving—the driver has the illusion that he or she can drive just fine while texting. Distracted eating is no different (Brunstrom and Mitchell 2006; Robinson et al. 2013). You might have the impression that you are aware of what you are putting in your mouth while reading the news or responding to e-mail. But you are truly missing out on the sensory aspects of eating—the sound of the crunch of lettuce, the cool silkiness of the sour cream next to the thick richness of a bean chili, the scent of cinnamon wafting from your oatmeal, or the visual tapestry of a colorful pasta salad. Although you have the ability to multitask, your mind can truly pay attention to only one thing at a time, like a camera lens. Consequently, if you are preoccupied with doing other activities while eating, not only will your enjoyment of your meal be diminished but also it is likely that you will not sense your fullness until you discover that you are too full and that you ate more than you needed. Or you might discover that you feel full, but because you didn't experience all the pleasures of your meal, you may still have a profound desire to continue eating to experience those joys.

Barriers to Fullness: Eating Without Distraction Self-Assessment

1. Place an X next to any of the activities that you frequently engage in while eating:

   ☐ watching television or a movie

   ☐ texting

   ☐ reading a book

   ☐ reading a magazine

   ☐ surfing the Internet

   ☐ reading or posting on social media

   ☐ working at your desk

☐ performing household chores

☐ sorting through your mail

☐ checking e-mail or voicemail

☐ checking your smartphone

☐ playing digital games

☐ creating to-do lists

☐ reading the newspaper

☐ reading the text on the cereal box

☐ walking around

☐ driving

☐ talking on the phone

☐ making your kids' lunches for school

☐ other: _____

2. Review the items that you checked off, then consider how often you engage in any kind of distracted eating?

☐ Every meal

☐ Most meals

☐ Only breakfast

☐ Only lunch

☐ Only dinner

☐ Only snacks

3. Think back at when you engaged in these activities while eating. In which cases do you remember being noticeably distracted from your food?

_____

_____

_____

4. What fears or thoughts of discomfort arise for you (if any), when you think about what it would be like to eat without engaging in any distracting activities?

_____

_____

_____

5. What do you need in order to feel ready to eat without distraction? Perhaps you have to ensure that you have enough time, that you have to eat in a room away from your television or computer, or that you have to come to an agreement with family members or roommates about it.

_____

_____

_____

6. Optimally, it would be important to avoid any activity that could distract you from the sensual qualities of eating, but that's usually too big of a step for most people. Describe one step you could take for eating without distraction. For example: *I will eat without distraction at several of my dinner meals for one week.*

_____

_____

Eating as Sacred Time: Create the Optimal Eating Environment

Whether you eat alone or with other people, eating is a time to connect with your body and nourish it, especially in regular meals (though the satisfaction and comfort of having a snack should not be seen as inconsequential). If you are with family, friends, or coworkers, it's also a time to connect with other people. But connection is difficult when there is unwanted distraction. It's important to create as optimal an eating experience as possible: pleasant, relaxed, and free from distraction. There are two key ways to do this: by setting boundaries and by creating a pleasant environment. Review the statements listed below and place a check by the ideas that you would be willing to try.

Set Boundaries	Create a Pleasant Environment
☐ Turn off all electronics, including those being used by other family members, with an exception made for music in the background. Unless absolutely necessary, don't answer the phone during meals.	☐ Designate one spot for eating, such as the kitchen or dining room table.
☐ Establish the expectation that meal times are not the place to hash out disagreements.	☐ Set a regular place setting—with a plate, utensils, and a napkin.
☐ Eat while sitting, not standing.	☐ Create a pleasant ambience by playing music, lighting a candle, or putting flowers on the table.

Clean Plate Club

Finishing all the food on your plate, regardless of how much is served, is an externally based pattern of eating and a barrier to experiencing fullness, disconnecting you from your internal body cues. Instead, your stopping point is when your plate is empty, regardless of your initial hunger and subsequent fullness level. This type of eating is also common with packages of food—eating until completion, until the package is empty. The familiar parental rule from childhood evolves into a habitual pattern and even an expectation. Other factors can trigger finishing all the food on your plate, including being too hungry, eating too fast, or fear of deprivation.

CLEAN PLATE ASSESSMENT

The next set of questions will help you evaluate tendencies to finish all the food on your plate and how to work with this habitual pattern, which does not serve the Intuitive Eating process.

1. Read the statements below, and check off the clean plate factors that resonate with you.

    ☐ I grew up in a large family, and meals were competitive. My mom put all the food on the table. If I didn't seize my servings, I lost out—there would be no food left.

    ☐ I grew up with a sense of food scarcity. Sometimes, I didn't know if there would be a next meal, so I made a point of eating *everything*.

☐ Sometimes there was just enough food served, and you were expected to eat it all.

☐ When I sit down to meals, I am usually ravenously hungry, and I have a high sense of urgency to eat—and to eat very fast.

☐ Finishing all the food on my plate was a value with which I was raised. It was considered wasteful to leave any food on my plate.

☐ When I am served a whole food, such as a sandwich, I automatically eat the entire thing.

☐ When I eat a package of food, such as potato chips, I automatically eat the entire package.

☐ I feel guilty if I don't eat all of my food.

☐ When I am in a restaurant, I tend to overeat to get my money's worth from the meal.

☐ When I am eating at an all-you-can-eat buffet, I tend to fill my plate and go back for more servings, even if I am full, in order to get my money's worth.

☐ When I was growing up, I had to finish all the food on my plate in order to get dessert.

☐ I eat very fast and typically finish eating before everybody else at the table.

☐ I worry about hurting people's feelings if they prepared a meal and expect me to eat it, even if I am too full.

2. Review the clean plate factors that affect you and answer the following questions:

A. What percentage of the time do you clean your plate?

☐ Rarely

☐ Less than half of my meals

☐ More than half of my meals

☐ All of my meals

B. Does cleaning your plate feel more like _____?

☐ An automatic habit

☐ A value (Note: if you experience guilt for leaving some food on your plate, it is likely part of your belief system or a personal value.)

C. If you are a clean plate eater, how difficult would it be for you to leave just one or two bites of food on your plate, if you become full before you have finished everything?

☐   Not at all difficult

☐   Somewhat difficult

☐   Very difficult

3. Practice Activity. To break the tendency of automatically eating all the food on your plate or from a package, try leaving one or two bites of food uneaten. The purpose of doing this is to break the habit of eating without regard for your satiety level. Practicing this technique will help you to create the pauses that will be needed in order to assess your fullness levels in the upcoming activities.

AUTOMATIC HABIT DISRUPTER: LEFT HAND EATING EXPERIMENT

A strong habit like cleaning your plate or eating fast may be insensitive to fullness cues because it is so conditioned and ingrained. But when habit automaticity is disrupted, it's easier for you to follow through with your intentions, such as leaving food on your plate when you become comfortably full. This next activity offers a novel way to disrupt the autopilot nature of these habits, which will enable you to savor the food and ultimately to be more connected to the physical sensations of emerging fullness.

The following technique is based on a clever study, in which subjects were merely asked to eat with their nondominant hand while watching a movie (Neal et al. 2011). In the first part of the study, the subjects ate with their dominant hand, and they were minimally influenced by their state of hunger or the palatability of the popcorn. (They were given equal amounts of *stale* and fresh popcorn and didn't notice the inferior popcorn.) In the second part of the study, the subjects were given a special popcorn box, which was constructed with a vertically aligned handle on one side. To prevent the subjects from using their dominant hand, they were instructed to slide the dominant hand between the handle and the box and hold the box in that manner throughout the movie. The result: less popcorn was eaten, especially if it was stale, because the subjects were more aware of what they were doing; their actions were no longer automatic.

So in the following activity, you will be eating with your nondominant hand (the left hand for most people). This activity is best performed in the privacy of your home. You will need to do something to ensure that you don't unconsciously begin using your dominant hand, such as strap it to your leg or waist with a belt. You can also simply slip it under your thigh or hold it behind your back while eating, but you will need to stay very aware of it. You should perform this experiment at a meal when you will not be interrupted and when you will have plenty of time to eat.

Eat your meal with your nondominant hand and take note of

- the sensations of emerging fullness as you eat, and

- the speed at which you are eating.

After you complete the experiment, answer the following questions:

1. How long did it take you to eat your meal? How similar or different was the duration of your meal compared to your usual meals?

_____

_____

_____

2. Was it easier to identify the sensations of emerging fullness? At what point during the meal did you begin to experience this?

_____

_____

_____

3. What would your eating be like if you were able to eat like this—at this speed and with these same sensations of fullness—when you were using your dominant hand?

_____

_____

_____

LEARNING TO SAY NO

In social settings, it's common for people to offer you more to eat. Sometimes a host is just being polite and accommodating, but some individuals gain self-worth from other people eating their food, especially if it is a special recipe. However, it's important for you to honor your body. It is not your responsibility to make someone happy by eating more food at the expense of your body and comfort. Even if they ask you repeatedly, if you don't want more to eat, you don't need to change your answer. Here are some ways you can politely say no to another offer of food. Place a check by the statements that resonate with you.

1.	No, thank you.
2.	I would love to eat more food, but I couldn't possibly have another bite without feeling uncomfortably full.
3.	Your dessert [or whatever the food is] looks delicious, but I am really too full to eat anything else. But I would love to take some home with me if there is any left over.
4.	No. Thank you. Really.
5.	Wow, your dish looks amazing. I am really too full to try it, but I would love to get the recipe from you, if you are willing to share it.
6.	I just ate dinner and did not realize you would be serving a meal at your party! Everything looks delicious, but I am really too full to eat anything else. But I would be happy to take a doggie bag if you have too many leftovers.
7.	I really appreciate that you made my favorite dish. It looks so yummy, and I know you spent a lot of time making it. I would really like to eat this when I can savor and enjoy it, but I'm just too full right now.
8.	No, thank you, again. But I would not feel good physically if I eat any more of your delicious food. I don't think you would want me to feel ill.
9.	Even just one more bite of food is too much for my body right now. Thank you for respecting my wish to stay comfortable.
10.	Yes, it's true that I usually say yes to your offers of more food. But I'm really working on listening to my body, for my health and comfort. And I have had enough to eat, thank you.

Helpful Tip: Make your decision to stop eating a conscious act. If you tend to be a clean plate eater, and you are eating with other people, you may wish to reinforce your decision to stop eating by doing something to make it a conscious act, such as putting your utensils on your plate. This simple act will help to prevent unintentional nibbling on the remaining food.

Characteristics of Fullness

There are many ways people experience fullness. Here are some of the different ways that you might experience signs of fullness during and after a meal. Check the statements that apply to you.

- ☐ Stomach: Many people experience a sensation of fullness in their stomach, ranging from a slight distention to heaviness and bloating.

- ☐ Head: Many experience fewer thoughts about food and eating. The desire to eat is diminished.

- ☐ Mood: Many feel a mood shift; they begin to feel pleasant or relaxed.

- ☐ Energy: Some people feel reenergized. Others, however; feel drowsy after eating.

- ☐ Other:_____

The Emergence of Fullness

Some people stop eating when they suddenly feel uncomfortably full. This sudden onset of extreme fullness arises from not paying attention to the emerging sensations of fullness. These sensations are subtle and easy to miss if you do not check in with your body. For many people, this requires slowing down the process of eating. The following activities will help you identify the sensations of fullness.

INTEROCEPTIVE AWARENESS WITH A WATER-DRINKING ACTIVITY

If you have been eating with distraction, it can cultivate a dissociative-like state, in which you are behaviorally eating, but your mind has left your body. Instead of paying attention to the sensations of eating, the mind is paying attention to another activity, such as watching television. In this situation, the emerging sensation of fullness can seem like a mystery unless it is profoundly unpleasant. In chapter 2, Honor Your Hunger, we discussed interoceptive awareness, the ability to perceive the physical sensations that arise within your body. Interoceptive awareness requires your attention.

Research shows that a specific water-drinking activity, called the *standardized water load test*, can help you identify the sensation of the stomach distension that is commonly associated with fullness (Herbert et al. 2012). It has been shown to be a valid indicator for the perception of fullness in both healthy people and in people with gastrointestinal disorders. This is one way to practice the perception of the physical sensations related to fullness. We want to emphasize the purpose of the activity is to connect to fullness sensations—it is *not* intended to trick your body into feeling full. (Besides, your body is too smart for that. When tricked into feeling full with a large amount of water, it will eventually recognize the deceit and resume indicating that it needs nourishment.)

Water-Drinking Activity

For this exercise, you will need two to four cups of noncarbonated water, at room temperature, and a five-minute period of time without interruption or distraction. When you are ready, begin drinking the water. There is no need to rush or guzzle the water.

- Notice the physical sensations of swallowing the water and water traveling down your esophagus.

- Don't stop drinking until you feel the first signs of fullness.

When you have recognized the sensation of fullness, answer the following questions.

1. Approximately how much water did you drink? _____

2. Describe the sensations of swallowing the water and having it travel down your esophagus.

   _____

   _____

   _____

3. How are these sensations similar to or different from the experience of fullness when eating food?

   _____

   _____

   _____

Practice the water-drinking activity as often as you need to in order to become familiar with perceiving the physical sensations associated with fullness.

Factors That Influence Fullness

There are several factors that influence how much food it takes for you to experience comfortable fullness.

- *Your Initial Hunger Level.* If you start eating when you're not hungry, there's no compass for the contrast of fullness, because there's no hunger to compare it to.

- *Unconditional Permission to Eat with Attunement.* If you have not made full peace with food (principle 3), then stopping because of fullness may seem like a difficult proposition. It's hard to stop eating if you believe you will never eat a particular food again.

- *Timing.* The amount of time that has passed since your last meal or snack will influence your fullness levels. To keep your energy and blood sugar in balance, you generally need to eat every two to six hours.

- *Amount of Food.* The amount of food that you ate at a prior meal or snack will influence when you become hungry and how much food it will take to reach comfortable fullness.

- *Social Influence.* Several studies have shown that the presence of people at a meal tends to increase the amount of food you eat. This may be due to distraction, peer pressure, or just simple unawareness.

- *Type of Food.* The kind of food you eat will influence not only your fullness level but also its staying power. For example, foods with a lot of bulk will make you feel full, but if they are also low in calories, such as vegetables or air-popped popcorn, they will not be satiating. Foods higher in fat, such as avocado, have more sustaining power. The next activity explores this issue in more depth.

Discovering the Fullness and Staying Power of Foods

It's helpful to be aware of how different types of foods affect your fullness level.

FOODS THAT INCREASE FULLNESS

Some types of foods contribute to the feeling of comfortable fullness:

Protein. The protein level in your meals or snacks helps to increase satiety levels. Foods high in protein include meats, beans, poultry, nuts, yogurt, and fish.

Fats. Fats contribute to fullness in two ways. First, the presence of fat in a meal slows down the rate of digestion. Fat is also the slowest part of food to be digested. It plays a significant role in prolonging fullness. Foods high in fats include nuts, salad dressings, oils, butter, nut butters, full-fat dairy products, and avocados.

Carbohydrates. Carbohydrates add bulk, which contributes to satiety. These foods also help to keep a normal blood sugar level, which is essential for providing energy to your cells. Foods high in carbohydrates include pasta, bread, rice, beans, and fruit.

Fiber. Fiber is an indigestible type of carbohydrate, which adds bulk and slows the absorption of carbohydrates into the blood stream. It's the reason a sandwich made with whole wheat bread may be a little more satisfying than one made with white bread, which has less fiber.

FOODS WITH LITTLE STAYING POWER

These type of foods temporarily contribute to the feeling of fullness, but it is a short-lived fullness, because they are low-calorie foods. It's the reason why, for example, you could eat a meal consisting of a big veggie salad (sans dressing and croutons), with a tall glass of unsweetened iced tea, and truly feel full, but then end up hungry only an hour or two later. Or you may have experienced a confusing feeling when eating these foods—you feel physically full, yet still feel like you are missing something. You feel like you are on the prowl, still needing to eat. Our patients often describe it as a restless, food-seeking feeling—they are not satisfied.

High Bulk, Low Calorie. These types of foods are generally vegetables and some fruits.

"Air Foods." These types of foods are usually familiar to dieters. Air foods fill up your stomach but offer little, if any, energy (calories). They are typically diet foods, such as rice cakes, puffed cereal, and sugar-free beverages.

Artificially Sweetened Foods and Low Carbohydrate Foods. These foods tend to replace carbohydrates with sugar-alcohols and indigestible fibers. These replacements can make you feel temporarily full (and if eaten in excess, they can cause bloating and discomfort). This includes some energy bars, sugar-free gelatin, and low-carbohydrate desserts and snack foods.

SATIETY SNACK PRACTICES

In order to experience how different foods affect your fullness level, over the next couple of days, choose at least one of the paired eating experiments below to try out. Be sure to try this at a time when you are experiencing hunger. It would also be best to make your other meals as identical as possible on those days (eating the same things and eating at the same time each day), so a more filling breakfast or a later lunch won't affect how filling the snack is. Under those controlled conditions, try a fruit smoothie one day and a peanut butter and jelly sandwich the next for comparison.

Paired Snack Options

1	Fruit Smoothie	versus	Peanut Butter and Jelly Sandwich
2	Special K Cereal with Milk	versus	Toast with Peanut Butter
3	Old-Fashioned Oatmeal	versus	Puffed Rice Cereal
4	Handful of Raisins	versus	Handful of Almonds
5	Energy Bar	versus	Nonfat Latte
6	Apple	versus	Apple with Peanut Butter
7	Nut Butter on Whole Wheat Bread	versus	Nut Butter on White Bread
8	Glass of Milk	versus	Glass of Juice
9	Cheese and Whole Grain Crackers	versus	Cheese and Rice Cakes
10	Granola Bar	versus	Greek Yogurt and Berries

Snack Satiety Experiment

Jot down the pair of snacks you plan to eat for comparison. Circle the amount of hours that the snack sustained you until you got hungry again.

Pair of Snacks Selected	Reoccurrence of Hunger (hours later)
Example—Snack A: Fruit Smoothie	0.5 1.5 2.0 2.5 3.0 3.5 4.0 4.5 5.0 5.5
Example—Snack B: Peanut Butter and Jelly Sandwich	0.5 1.5 2.0 2.5 3.0 3.5 4.0 4.5 5.0 5.5
	0.5 1.5 2.0 2.5 3.0 3.5 4.0 4.5 5.0 5.5
	0.5 1.5 2.0 2.5 3.0 3.5 4.0 4.5 5.0 5.5
	0.5 1.5 2.0 2.5 3.0 3.5 4.0 4.5 5.0 5.5
	0.5 1.5 2.0 2.5 3.0 3.5 4.0 4.5 5.0 5.5

REFLECTION

Describe one of the snack experiments you tried. What did you expect to happen?

_____

_____

Which snack lasted for a longer period of time before you got hungry again?

_____

_____

Why do you think a particular snack sustained you for a longer period of time?

_____

_____

How can you apply what you discovered to your snacks for making them more sustainable (if desired)?

_____

_____

DISCOVERING MEALS WITH STAYING POWER

Let's build upon what you have learned about the staying power of snacks and apply it to your meals. In addition to evaluating the sustaining qualities of a meal, you will also be paying attention to how the sensation of fullness wanes after eating a meal.

On the following worksheet, choose a few of your favorite or typical meals over the week to rate. In order to gauge how long the feeling of fullness lasts, you will rate your fullness every thirty minutes, for the two-hour period, after a meal. In the last column, note how long it took until you became hungry again (this could be from one to six hours later).

Getting to Know Fullness Worksheet

Meal (Note the date, time, and type, and approximate amount of food.)	Duration of Fullness after Meal (minutes)	Rate Fullness (0–10)	Reoccurrence of Hunger (hours later)
	30 minutes	0 1 2 3 4 5 6 7 8 9 10	
	60 minutes	0 1 2 3 4 5 6 7 8 9 10	
	90 minutes	0 1 2 3 4 5 6 7 8 9 10	
	120 minutes	0 1 2 3 4 5 6 7 8 9 10	
	30 minutes	0 1 2 3 4 5 6 7 8 9 10	
	60 minutes	0 1 2 3 4 5 6 7 8 9 10	
	90 minutes	0 1 2 3 4 5 6 7 8 9 10	
	120 minutes	0 1 2 3 4 5 6 7 8 9 10	
	30 minutes	0 1 2 3 4 5 6 7 8 9 10	
	60 minutes	0 1 2 3 4 5 6 7 8 9 10	
	90 minutes	0 1 2 3 4 5 6 7 8 9 10	
	120 minutes	0 1 2 3 4 5 6 7 8 9 10	
	30 minutes	0 1 2 3 4 5 6 7 8 9 10	
	60 minutes	0 1 2 3 4 5 6 7 8 9 10	
	90 minutes	0 1 2 3 4 5 6 7 8 9 10	
	120 minutes	0 1 2 3 4 5 6 7 8 9 10	

REFLECTION

Review your Getting to Know Fullness Worksheet and then answer the following questions.

What types of meals helped to sustain your fullness level? For how long?

_____

_____

What types of foods did you eat that did not sustain you for several hours (that is, you were hungry again too soon after the meal)?

_____

_____

Based on your experiences, describe the components of a meal that would sustain you for several hours.

_____

_____

Describe the trend of your fullness levels when you checked in every thirty minutes for a two-hour period after a meal.

_____

_____

Describe any surprises or unexpected experiences with getting to know fullness from meals.

_____

_____

FULLNESS DISCOVERY SCALE

In order to really get dialed in to the nuances of your fullness, you will need a lot of practice listening for it. Using the Fullness Discovery Scale Journal that follows (and is available for download at http://www.newharbinger.com/26224), keep track of your hunger rating and fullness rating, the quality of the fullness, and the foods eaten for a meal or snack. Do try to be accurate with the time that you ate, as it will help you to see any patterns and trends with your intensity of hunger between meals. Do this for several days. (You may want to make copies of the journal.)

In the journal, first, rate your hunger by circling the number that best reflects your hunger level before your meal or snack. Then begin to eat, but pause in the middle of your snack or meal and gauge (1) the taste of the food, and (2) any sensations of diminishing hunger and emerging fullness. Finally, when you have had enough to eat, rate your fullness level from 0 to 10. Note the quality of your fullness level: is it pleasant, unpleasant, or neutral? In the last column, note if you were doing another activity simultaneously while you were eating (such as reading, surfing the Internet, texting, and so forth).

Fullness Discovery Scale Journal

Time	Hunger Rating	Fullness Rating	Quality of Fullness			Meal or Food Eaten	Simultaneous Activity?
			Pleasant	Unpleasant	Neutral		
	0 1 2 3 4 5 6 7 8 9 10	0 1 2 3 4 5 6 7 8 9 10					
	0 1 2 3 4 5 6 7 8 9 10	0 1 2 3 4 5 6 7 8 9 10					
	0 1 2 3 4 5 6 7 8 9 10	0 1 2 3 4 5 6 7 8 9 10					
	0 1 2 3 4 5 6 7 8 9 10	0 1 2 3 4 5 6 7 8 9 10					
	0 1 2 3 4 5 6 7 8 9 10	0 1 2 3 4 5 6 7 8 9 10					

REFLECTION ON YOUR FULLNESS RATINGS

Review your satiety ratings and look for trends and patterns. Then answer the following questions.

At which point did you usually feel the sensations of fullness? Perhaps at a 6, perhaps at an 8?

_____

_____

_____

By the time you stopped eating because of fullness, did your fullness experience tend to be pleasant, unpleasant, or neutral?

_____

_____

What trends did you notice between your hunger and fullness ratings? For example, if you began eating with an unpleasantly hungry rating of a 2 or less, did it take eating more food to experience fullness?

_____

_____

If you engaged in another activity while eating, what impact did it have on your fullness rating?

_____

_____

What types of foods did you eat that helped you to become comfortably full?

_____

_____

Were there any meals in which it took more than the usual amount of food to feel full? If yes, was there any relationship to your initial hunger level or any simultaneous activity you were engaged in?

_____

_____

THE LAST BITE THRESHOLD

As you begin to become more familiar with the various sensations of fullness, you will be able to identify the *last bite threshold*, which is the endpoint of eating (for now). It's a subtle experience. You become aware that just one more bite of food will likely be your stopping point for a comfortable satiety level. The key element in sensing this threshold is paying attention. On that front, you already have some nice experience under your belt, since you have practiced the fullness exercises in this chapter. For most people, paying enough attention to fullness to sense the last bite threshold will take more practice and patience. There are some specific steps that can help you increase your awareness of the last bite threshold:

- When you finish eating, reflect on how you feel physically. Really check in and notice the sensations of your fullness. Linger with these sensations for a few minutes.

- Next ask yourself, *How would I feel if I had stopped a few bites sooner?* Note the thoughts that arise. Perhaps you notice a curiosity and desire to explore this idea at your next meal. Maybe that idea is threatening to you. Perhaps the idea makes you sad. That's okay. Just notice these feelings, without judgment, and jot down your thoughts here:

_____

_____

_____

_____

If you feel ready to experiment with stopping at a few bites sooner, move on to the next activity, the Last Bite Threshold Experiment. In order to meaningfully complete this experiment, you need to be at a place where you can recognize general fullness. If you are not at that point yet, that's okay. It simply means that you need more practice working with the Fullness Discovery Scale Journal. Remember that becoming an Intuitive Eater is not a race, and it is important to work at a pace that feels comfortable for you.

Last Bite Threshold Experiment

Select a meal that will be relaxed and free of distraction.

1. Using the techniques described in the instructions for the Fullness Discovery Scale Journal, take a prolonged pause when you are at the point of detecting the absence of hunger and the emergence of fullness (that's step 2).

2. Estimate roughly how many more bites of food it will take to be comfortably full (note that you don't need to estimate an exact number of bites). And tentatively mark that as your stopping point.

3. Continue eating with profound awareness with each bite of food.

   • Notice how the food feels in your mouth and tastes.

   • After swallowing, notice how your body feels.

   • Before taking the next bite of food, ask yourself, is it possible that this next bite is the last bite for me? If your gut sense is yes, plan to stop at that point.

4. Notice how you feel. It may be important to remind yourself that you can still eat the rest of this particular food or meal again. Remember there are no forbidden foods.

The more you practice this activity, the more adept you will become at recognizing the last bite threshold. Reflect on your experience.

_____

_____

_____

_____

Wrap-Up

In this chapter, you learned different ways to become connected to the sensation of fullness and how to overcome barriers to responding to this cue in a timely and meaningful manner. You discovered a number of factors that affect satiety, including the other people present when you are eating, the time you last ate, the types of foods you are eating, and your initial hunger level. In the next chapter, you will discover the importance of the satisfaction factor in eating, which is the hub of the Intuitive Eating principles.

CHAPTER 6

Principle Six
Discover the Satisfaction Factor

The Japanese have the wisdom to promote pleasure as one of their goals of healthy living. In our fury to be thin and healthy, we often overlook one of the most basic gifts of existence—the pleasure and satisfaction that can be found in the eating experience. When you eat what you really want, in an environment that is inviting and conducive, the pleasure you derive will be a powerful force in helping you feel satisfied and content. By providing this experience for yourself, you will find that it takes much less food to decide you've had enough.

Why Satisfaction and Pleasure Are Important

Nothing would be more tiresome than eating and drinking if God had not made them a pleasure as well as a necessity.

—Voltaire

Unfortunately, for so many in our culture, the pleasure of eating promotes feelings of guilt and wrongdoing, and, of course, dieting plays right into this ethic. It causes you to make sacrifices and settle for less. But if you regularly settle for an unsatisfying food or an unappetizing eating experience, satisfaction will not be the outcome; rather, you are likely to continue searching for a satisfying food, even though you are no longer hungry. Fortunately, studies show that Epicurean eating pleasure—a concept that involves an ongoing appreciation of the aesthetics of foods, their symbolic value, and the pursuit of pleasure—is correlated with smaller portions and higher well-being, yet is not associated with higher body mass index (Cornil and Chandon 2015). Eat what is truly satisfying and pleasurable, without attaching morality, and achieve increased psychological and biological health! It is no wonder that the French, who revere the pleasure of eating, have the third lowest rate of heart disease in the world.

Satisfaction is the hub of the wheel of Intuitive Eating. It is the touchstone for all of the Intuitive Eating principles (see figure 6.1). Each principle promotes your ability to find the most satisfaction in your meal. You will find that eating when you are moderately hungry, rather than ravenous or not hungry at all, will ensure more satisfaction. When you eat without a diet mentality, while making peace with food and challenging the food police, you'll be free to discover satisfaction. You will receive more pleasure from a meal that is eaten without emotional turmoil. Respect for your body comes with an appreciation for the wonders of your body's many capacities, including the enjoyment of food. Moving your body regularly and eating with an intention to feel good physically allows for far more satisfaction in life in general—and especially in eating.

Satisfaction: The Hub of Intuitive Eating

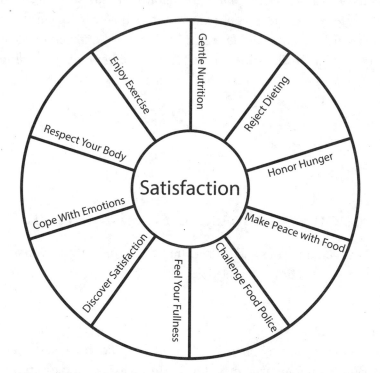

Figure 6.1.   Satisfaction: The Hub of Intuitive Eating.
Reprinted with permission from Tribole and Resch 2012 / St. Martin's Press.

Keep in mind that honoring each of the Intuitive Eating principles will give you the best chance of achieving the greatest satisfaction in your meals. In this chapter, you will be offered exercises to help you better understand this connection, so that you may regain your satisfaction and pleasure in eating.

What Do You Really Want to Eat?

In order to feel satisfied when eating, the first question to ask is, "What do I *really* want to eat?" This may be difficult for you, if you have never been asked about what you liked or wanted to eat. Begin by exploring your childhood eating experiences by answering the following questions:

- Did your parent or caregiver give you any choices in terms of what you were served?

- Was there a diet mentality or an extreme focus on eating only healthy food?

- Were there good foods and bad foods and even forbidden foods in your home?

- Were you punished if you did not follow the household food rules?

- Was it stressful to eat around your family members? Perhaps they were overly critical of your food choices.

_____

_____

_____

_____

Sensory Considerations

Respect your taste buds' preferences. You may have true life-long preferences or dislikes for certain tastes or foods, but it's important to consider that your tastes may change over time. You may have gotten caught up in a rebellious food fight, thinking that you didn't like certain foods, and be surprised to find that you now like them. As an Intuitive Eater, be committed to choosing the foods that you truly enjoy, without applying moralistic judgment. Remember, only you can know what pleases and satisfies your taste buds. Don't settle—if you don't love it, don't eat it, and if you love it, savor it!

The following questions will help you identify what it is you truly want to eat. It is most helpful to answer these questions when you are moderately hungry—perhaps a 3 or a 4 on the Description of Hunger and Fullness Sensations chart in chapter 2. As you go through the sensory considerations, ask yourself what feels right to you in this moment.

WHAT TASTE SOUNDS APPEALING?

Consider these taste qualities: savory, sweet, salty, buttery, rich, bitter, tart, smoky, hot and spicy, bland, or mild.

Would something primarily sweet, such as a yam or a cookie, offer you satisfaction? Consider the following questions: Was your last meal primarily sweet? Did you have something like sweetened cereal and a piece of toast with jelly for breakfast? Would your enjoyment of the sweet flavor of the foods you've already eaten inform the flavor you'd like to experience right now?

_____

_____

Think about foods that are salty—a pickle, for example—or perhaps a savory flavor, like pasta with a rich tomato sauce. Imagine that salty or savory taste on your tongue. Does it feel right to you at this moment?

_____

_____

Now think about foods that are mild and even bland, perhaps cottage cheese and fruit. Imagine that mild flavor on your tongue and in your body. Is this the right flavor for you right now?

_____

_____

Is there another flavor sensation that appeals to you?

_____

_____

WHAT TEXTURE SOUNDS INTERESTING?

Consider these textures which a food or meal offers: smooth, creamy, crunchy, chewy, crispy, crumbly, hard, soft, flaky, gooey, mushy, sticky, greasy, dry, moist, thick, thin, heavy, light, or lumpy.

1. Imagine the sensation of a smooth, silky food, such as pudding, on your tongue.

2. Now, think about eating something crunchy. Would you like to crunch on lettuce leaves in a salad or perhaps some corn chips?

3. Maybe smooth or crunchy don't appeal to you right now, but something chewy is more desirable. Perhaps a steak or a bagel would give you that sensation.

4. Is there another texture that's more appealing?

5. Perhaps you want a variety of textures in this meal.

6. You might find that none of these textures fits the bill in this moment and that you'd rather have the experience of drinking without chewing. Then a smoothie might do it.

What texture would you like right now?

_____

_____

What food or foods would provide that texture?

_____

_____

WHAT DISTINCT AROMAS ARE APPEALING?

Much of the pleasure of eating comes from smelling. People who have a diminished sense of smell receive much less pleasure when they eat. Each of the foods you identified above for its appealing tastes and textures may also have a distinct aroma that may or may not be appealing to you.

In this moment, is there an aroma that comes to mind that would spark your palate?

- Does the smell of roasted garlic or onions, sizzling bacon, grilled steak, or pizza heating in the oven appeal to you?

- Or would the aroma of hot coffee, cinnamon, or vanilla be just right?

- Or buttery popcorn or fresh-baked bread?

- What about a smelly cheese or something smoky, fishy, or lemony?

_____

_____

WHAT TEMPERATURE OF FOOD IS ENTICING?

Another sensory consideration is the temperature of food. Imagine being inside the house while it's raining and cold outside. You may be sitting in front of a roaring fire and reading a good book when your first hunger signals emerge.

Does a bowl of steaming soup seem right at that moment? _____

Now, imagine that you're lying on a lounge chair on the beach on a hot summer day, watching the ocean waves breaking.

A bowl of soup may not fit in this scenario. Does a cold milkshake or a cool bowl of fresh fruit with cottage cheese feel perfect?

_____

Consider the temperature of your beverages in making your meal more satisfying.

If you want coffee, would you prefer it hot or more tepid? _____

Or, perhaps, would you like tea, either iced or hot? _____

If you're drinking water, would you prefer it with ice or at room temperature?

_____

WHAT ABOUT THE APPEARANCE OF FOOD?

The look of the food on your plate can affect how satisfying your eating experience will be. Experiment with the following image of a chicken dinner. Visualize a plate filled with a poached chicken breast whose skin looks barely cooked. Next to it is steamed cauliflower and some mashed potatoes. Is this beige meal appealing to you? Does this image provide a pleasurable meal? Now, transform that meal by considering color. The chicken is roasted to a golden brown color. Replace the cauliflower with grilled asparagus spears, and replace the mashed potatoes with yams topped with a bit of cinnamon. Disregarding how much you like or dislike the actual foods on the two plates, consider how much these changes to the mere appearance of the meal change your enthusiasm for eating it.

When you think about what you really want to eat, ask the following questions:

Would I like something colorful and diverse or uncomplicated and bland looking?

_____

How would any of these appearances affect the satisfaction of your meal?

_____

_____

Some other aspects of food appearance could be vertical height, such as a tower of food; flat, like a quesadilla; different textures and shapes and sizes of items on the plate; and the arrangement of food (all in one bowl or on separate plates, like an assortment of appetizers or items on a buffet table).

HOW DO YOU FEEL ABOUT THE VOLUME AND SUSTAINING CAPACITY OF THE FOOD?

The last sensual quality to examine is the volume of food, which will be experienced in your stomach rather than through your senses. Some foods, like a hearty bean chili, digest slowly. If you eat a big salad or steamed vegetables, they'll fill you up right away but not give you much satiety, because they digest more quickly. When you're choosing what to eat, consider the following:

Do you want something heavy and hearty that will fill you up and that will sustain you for a long time, like macaroni and cheese or beef stew?

Or do you want something airy, light, or small, which might not fill your stomach or might not hold you very long, such as popcorn, yogurt, or an energy bar?

_____

_____

Now that you have considered the taste, texture, aroma, temperature, appearance, and volume of the potential foods you will choose for a meal, store these sensual considerations in your mind. Remember them each time you ask yourself, *What do I really want to eat right now?* Consider each of your senses. Then think about the meal as a whole. You may not be able to satisfy each of your senses in every meal. That's okay. Choose the components that are most important in the moment.

The Importance of Eating Slowly and Mindfully

Inner awareness, or mindfulness, is a critical part of the entire process of Intuitive Eating. Staying present allows you to feel the direct experience of your body and the many sensations of eating. To help you practice this mindfulness, we have developed the Intuitive Eating Awareness Training (iEAT).

iEAT Scripted Activity

This is a guided eating activity to help cultivate your awareness and experience of the many sensory nuances of eating, which will ultimately contribute to your satisfaction in eating.

GET READY

It would be helpful for you to read aloud the script (below) and record it—for instance, as a voice memo on your smartphone, which you can replay during the exercise, but be sure to turn the ringer off on your phone so you are not disturbed by a call. This will allow you to place all of your attention on the eating process (rather than trying to juggle the reading with your eating experience). Then follow these next five steps:

1. Select a time and a place in which you can eat without distraction.

2. Choose a small food that you would like to eat that does not require utensils (such as dried fruit, nuts, a pretzel, a piece of chocolate, a slice of bread, a small piece of fruit, some granola, or a cookie).

3. Provide a napkin or plate.

4. Turn off the ringer on your phone and other devices, including the sound of incoming texts.

5. Replay the recording you made of the script below and follow its instructions.

iEAT Script

Place your food on a plate or napkin in front of you. Sit comfortably in your chair and take a couple of deep breaths, until you feel relaxed and calm. It is important to take your time and not rush into each of the following experiences.

Sight. Without touching your food, notice how it looks on the plate or napkin. Gaze upon it with curiosity, as if you have never seen this type of food before. Notice the color, the shape, and any nooks and crannies and shadows. How would you describe what you observe to someone who has never seen this food? There is no wrong or right way to describe your observation. Just notice and engage your eyes.

Smell. Place your nose near the food and gently inhale. What does the food smell like? Is there a scent? Perhaps hints of vanilla, mint, chocolate, or a spicy or pungent aroma? Is the scent subtle or strong? Or perhaps the scent is fragrant but neither subtle nor strong? There is no wrong or right way to experience aroma. Just notice.

Touch. Pick up the food and place it in your hand. Notice how it feels in your hand. Perhaps it is smooth, rough, sharp, crumbly, sticky, brittle, crusty, heavy, or light? There is no wrong or right way to describe physical sensations of touch. Just notice and feel the texture.

Sound. Take a small bite of the food. How does it sound as you take a bite? Perhaps crunchy, crackly, dull, slurpy, or wispy? There is no wrong or right way to describe what you hear. Just listen and notice.

Mouthfeel. Without taking another bite, roll the food around in your mouth and notice how it feels. Is the texture rough, crumbly, dry, sticky, moist, light, or something else? Resist the urge to chew the food; just notice how the texture of the food changes as it sits on your tongue. Perhaps it's beginning to get soggy, to disintegrate, or to become stringy or sharp. There is no wrong or right way to describe physical sensations of food in your mouth. Just notice and feel the texture gradually change.

Taste. How does the food taste? Perhaps sweet, sour, bitter, salty, pungent, or bland? What happens to the taste of the food as it sits on your tongue? Does it get stronger, or perhaps more subtle and less distinct. Are new flavors emerging as the food dissolves on your tongue? There is no wrong or right way to taste your food. Just observe and notice the nuance of flavors.

Next, chew your bite of food and, when you feel ready, swallow it. Notice how the food feels as it travels down your throat. Take another bite of your food and repeat this process.

iEAT PRACTICE

Now that you have experienced paying attention to specific senses while eating, it's important to continue to practice this mindful eating. For this upcoming week, select six meals or snacks in which you can devote your attention to the sensory aspects of eating. Use the iEAT Practice Worksheet below to record these experiences. Pay attention to and check off all of your sensory experiences while eating a meal or snack, and then describe your experience.

iEAT Practice Worksheet

Date	Meal or Snack	Sensory Experience						Comments (Describe your sensory experience.)
		Sight	Smell	Touch	Sound	Taste	Mouthfeel	

iEAT REFLECTION

How did the iEAT experience compare with your usual process of eating? Consider the time spent eating and the different sensory experiences.

_____

_____

What would you need to do in order to eat in this manner with most of your meals? Consider setting an intention to select one meal, such as lunch, as you begin practicing this process.

_____

_____

How did paying attention to sensory aspects contribute to your satisfaction in eating?

_____

_____

ADVANCED iEAT PRACTICE: DISTRACTING THOUGHTS

Although you have been working at eating most of your meals without engaging in distracting behaviors (such as watching television, reading, or checking for text messages), you might still find yourself distracted by your thoughts. Perhaps you find yourself ruminating on a conversation that didn't go well with your boss, stressing about an upcoming deadline, or comparing your meal to your dining companion's meal. Distracting thoughts can pull you away from the experience and satisfaction of eating. One way to deal with this issue is a process involving two steps (which often need to be repeated):

- Select a sensory focal point for your meal, such as how a food tastes or perhaps its mouthfeel. Each time you notice yourself lost in thought while eating, simply label it as "thinking," without judgment.

- Gently direct your mind to the sensory focal point of your meal, such as paying attention to the taste or mouthfeel of the food.

Be prepared to repeat those two steps often. The real practice here is redirecting your mind to an eating focal point and away from your thoughts. This process is very similar to the process of simply noticing stray thoughts during meditation and gently bringing your attention back to your breath.

Sensory Specific Satiety

In the field of hedonics—the study of pleasure—the concept of pleasantness is important in influencing food choice and may play a role in determining the amount of food consumed. This is called sensory specific satiety (SSS). Studies of SSS have found that it occurs within two minutes after consumption of a single food, when there's been little opportunity for digestion and absorption, and it's specific for the sensory aspects of the food (Rolls 1986; Hetherington, Rolls, and Burley 1989). If you are eating mindfully, you will begin to notice when that moment of SSS sets in, for example, when your taste buds begin to be desensitized to the taste. At that moment, you might notice that it doesn't taste as good as it did when you first bit into it. SSS encompasses the proposition that by evaluating the sensual qualities of food, which you identified in the preceding exercise, you can determine when the pleasantness of food decreases. With this focus, you'll naturally come to just the right amount of food you need to give you the most satisfaction.

Typically, we eat more than one food in a meal. As the pleasantness of a group of foods decreases, it often corresponds to an increase in satiety, leading to a decrease in hunger and desire to eat.

Advanced Practice: Detecting Sensory Specific Satiety

For this exercise, first check in with your hunger to see if you're moderately hungry. Then pick one food that appeals to you, after going through all of your senses, as you did above (in the section What Do You Really Want to Eat?). Make sure you try this with only one food. Note the time. Begin to eat, slowly and mindfully. As you continue eating, ask yourself the following questions:

- Has the flavor diminished?

- Does it still smell as good?

- Is the texture and appearance still as appealing?

When you notice that the "pleasantness" of the food has lessened, note the time to see how many minutes have passed. How long did it take for SSS to set in?

_____

Repeat this exercise, but this time, serve yourself a meal with a variety of foods. Does it take longer for the pleasantness of the meal to diminish when there is a variety of foods? How many minutes?

_____

With this knowledge, you will find that by stopping at the point that the pleasantness of the food diminishes, you'll walk away from the meal, physically comfortable and satisfied. And don't worry—your body has wisdom; you'll get just the amount of nutrition that your body needs over time.

The Impact of Hunger and Fullness

Have you ever eaten very little during the day when you know that you'll be going out to a lovely dinner in the evening? People do this all of the time, saving up for the meal without considering the consequences. It's common to ignore the fact that going into a meal feeling ravenous is a sure route to gorging on as much food as you can to satisfy yourself. Once you're in a state of primal hunger, all possibility of true satisfaction from your meal is removed by the drive to get the food in quickly. Likewise, it is just as hard to be satisfied from a meal if you sit down to eat when you have no noticeable hunger at all. You will get more pleasure out of a meal that's begun when you're moderately hungry.

Last Bite Threshold

The *last bite threshold* is the point at which your body gives you the cue that you are at a comfortable fullness level (around 6 or 7 on the Hunger Discovery Scale in chapter 2). At this point, you will find that satisfaction in what you are eating will begin to diminish. For the greatest satisfaction, be sure to provide a variety of foods and to practice ending your meal when you reach physical satiety. The Satisfaction Discovery Worksheet will help you find the last bite threshold as you're rating your fullness.

Satisfaction Discovery Worksheet

Circle the number that best reflects your hunger level before your meal or snack. When finished eating, rate your fullness, and then rate your level of satisfaction. Remember, there is no right or wrong number; it's merely a method to help you listen to and discover satisfaction in eating. At this point, you will have found the last bite threshold.

Time	Hunger Rating	Food Eaten	Fullness Rating	Satisfaction Rating	Comments
	0 1 2 3 4 5 6 7 8 9 10		0 1 2 3 4 5 6 7 8 9 10	0 1 2 3 4 5 6 7 8 9 10	
	0 1 2 3 4 5 6 7 8 9 10		0 1 2 3 4 5 6 7 8 9 10	0 1 2 3 4 5 6 7 8 9 10	
	0 1 2 3 4 5 6 7 8 9 10		0 1 2 3 4 5 6 7 8 9 10	0 1 2 3 4 5 6 7 8 9 10	
	0 1 2 3 4 5 6 7 8 9 10		0 1 2 3 4 5 6 7 8 9 10	0 1 2 3 4 5 6 7 8 9 10	
	0 1 2 3 4 5 6 7 8 9 10		0 1 2 3 4 5 6 7 8 9 10	0 1 2 3 4 5 6 7 8 9 10	
	0 1 2 3 4 5 6 7 8 9 10		0 1 2 3 4 5 6 7 8 9 10	0 1 2 3 4 5 6 7 8 9 10	
	0 1 2 3 4 5 6 7 8 9 10		0 1 2 3 4 5 6 7 8 9 10	0 1 2 3 4 5 6 7 8 9 10	
	0 1 2 3 4 5 6 7 8 9 10		0 1 2 3 4 5 6 7 8 9 10	0 1 2 3 4 5 6 7 8 9 10	
	0 1 2 3 4 5 6 7 8 9 10		0 1 2 3 4 5 6 7 8 9 10	0 1 2 3 4 5 6 7 8 9 10	

© 2017 Evelyn Tribole / New Harbinger Publications

Reflection on the Satisfaction Discovery Worksheet

What trends did you notice with hunger, fullness, and satisfaction?

_____

_____

Did you notice the last bite threshold? If so, by identifying this point, were you able to hone your satisfaction quotient even more acutely?

_____

_____

In this section, you have learned and practiced that you will have the best chance of finding satisfaction in your meals when you begin eating with moderate hunger and eat to a point of comfortable fullness. At this point, you have reached the last bite threshold, which brings with it diminished pleasantness and satisfaction from the food you're eating.

Your Eating Environment

People frequently treat eating as they might treat washing their laundry—just going through the motions of a necessary but dull task, hardly paying attention—simply just getting through it. If you choose to eat your meals without regard to your environment, the satisfaction of eating can be diminished. The following exercises will help you create a peaceful and inviting environment that will maximize your satisfaction.

Examine Your Current Eating Environment

How much time do you allot for your meals? _____

Where do you eat most of your meals—at home, in a restaurant, at school, at work?

_____

Do you sit, stand, or walk while eating? _____

Are you engaged in other activities while eating, such as talking on the telephone, sitting in front of your computer, watching television, driving, or something else?

_____

Whom do you eat with—a friend, a partner or family members, work or school associates, or someone else? Or are you eating alone?

_____

If you're eating at home, do you eat at the dining room or kitchen table, or are you eating at your desk or on the couch? Is the area clear or cluttered?

_____

If you have a table, describe what it looks like. Does it appeal to your aesthetics? What kind of plates and utensils do you use? Are they paper, plastic, ceramic, stainless steel, or something else?

_____

_____

Do you play music while you eat? _____

Which emotions do you generally feel when you eat? Are you calm, anxious, bored, fearful, or something else?

_____

Reflection

What are your impressions of your current eating environment?

_____

_____

_____

_____

_____

Do you notice any themes or trends from your responses above?

_____

_____

_____

The Intuitive Eating Workbook

Consider these possible issues:

- *Time to Enjoy Eating.* You may be eating rapidly and trying to squeeze your mealtime into a five-minute slot between jobs or chores. Or are you giving yourself plenty of time to appreciate your food?

- *Distracted Eating.* If you are standing up while eating, whether it be in front of the refrigerator, looking out the window, or racing around the house, you are missing the opportunity to sit, relax, look at your food on the plate, and take in its sensual qualities. If you are engaging in these activities while eating, it is unlikely that you can focus on your meal.

- *People.* Eating with someone else can often enhance your pleasurable experience, but it can sometimes distract you from your food. If you're comparing what you're eating with another's meal, or you're engaged in an uncomfortable conversation, it's possible that you won't notice whether the food is actually to your liking or whether you're beginning to reach your last bite threshold. (Consider your companions at each meal. It may vary.)

- *Clutter.* If your eating space is cluttered, and there's barely room to set down your plate, the mess can distract you, and you will not have a calm, satisfying eating experience.

- *Setting.* If you eat in an unattractive setting, you're not honoring the experience of eating and not receiving the ultimate satisfaction that eating can offer.

- *Noise.* If you listen to loud, head-banging music, or there's construction going on next door, or your coworkers are arguing or talking loudly at the next cubicle, you will feel the antithesis of a soothing environment.

- *Stressful Emotions.* If your emotions are intense, it's difficult to feel calm enough to enjoy your meal.

Cultivating a Pleasant Eating Environment

If you create an intention to reduce as many distractions as you can, while increasing the pleasantness of your eating environment, then your chances of achieving satisfaction in your meals greatly increase.

What modifications could you make in your home to provide a more pleasant eating environment?

_____

_____

_____

_____

_____

Your Emotional Connection to Eating

For some, mealtime is a sacred time, set aside for enjoyment and pleasure. For others, it feels like a battleground or a prison.

Your Emotional Atmosphere

Contemplate the following questions:

How often is there chaos in your house when you begin to eat a meal? Chaos could include the dog barking, the baby crying, everyone rushing to get to work or school on time, a cluttered table, the phone ringing incessantly, and so on. What can you do to reduce some of this chaos? Perhaps you could get up fifteen minutes earlier to give yourself a moment to breathe and contemplate the gratitude you feel for some of the gifts in your life. Maybe you can turn the ringer off on the phone while you are eating and clear off the table the night before. Or if your timing allows, you might want to have a snack before you get the kids off to school and can then return home and sit down to enjoy your meal. What changes are you willing and able to make?

_____

_____

_____

Is the room (at home, at work, or at school) filled with tension? If there is tension between you and your partner, your parent, or any member of your household, take the brave step of finding a time outside of mealtime to speak up about what you're feeling and what you need. If possible, consider seeking counseling, either for yourself or group counseling with the others, to improve the emotional situation in your home.

_____

_____

_____

_____

Are people arguing during mealtime? If others are arguing among themselves and bringing that argument to the table, speak up and ask that they either resolve their problems at another time or refrain from engaging in them while eating. This is not your problem, but it affects your enjoyment of your meal. Set up a nonargument zone during meals. How will you do this?

_____

_____

_____

_____

Is there plenty of food available? Do you feel that you won't get enough to eat or that there won't be enough variety, so that you can choose what you actually feel like eating? If your refrigerator is bare, because neither you nor anyone else in your home has done the food shopping, develop a plan for who will do the shopping and a regular time for this to occur. What ideas do you have for resolving this situation?

_____

_____

_____

_____

Are people criticizing what or how much you eat? If they are, it's highly unlikely that you can focus on your enjoyment of your meal, since you're eating in a hostile environment. What boundaries can you set to create a neutral eating environment?

_____

_____

_____

You deserve to have an emotionally healthy and happy eating environment. You may not be able to accomplish all of them—certainly not at once—but each incremental step you can take will lead you to more pleasure and satisfaction in your eating.

Your Favorites: Foods, Dining Companions, and Places to Eat

Spending a moment contemplating your favorites—foods, places to eat, and companions—will increase the chances of enjoyable eating experiences.

What are your favorite foods?

_____

_____

_____

_____

Who are your favorite eating companions? If you eat with people whom you enjoy (including yourself ☺) and with whom you feel safe, your meals will be more satisfying.

_____

_____

_____

_____

Do you like to eat at home, in restaurants, at friends' homes, at parties, at large events, or in some other setting? List your favorite places to eat in order to heighten your satisfaction in your meals.

_____

_____

_____

_____

_____

The next time you are planning an outing involving eating, take some time to remember your favorites—special foods, people, and places. You'll find that the quality of your eating experience will be heightened.

Wrap-Up

Discovering the satisfaction factor of eating is a full mind-body experience. It allows you the freedom to pick just the right food for your taste buds. Be sure to stop trying to gain satisfaction from food that's not hitting the spot. It can have an unfortunate result. You might end up overeating and then looking for yet *another* food to satisfy yourself. Be sure to monitor any remnants of guilt you hold about your choice of food. They will diminish your eating experience.

In this chapter, you have evaluated what you really want to eat, as well as other factors geared toward getting the most satisfaction possible from your meals. Remember, it takes time and patience, and you must learn not to judge yourself. Practicing staying present is an important factor for achieving satisfaction in your eating. Doing so may be your first step in finding a more fulfilling life.

In the next chapter, you will delve more deeply into how to cope with your emotions without using food.

CHAPTER 7

Principle Seven
Cope with Your Feelings Without Using Food

Find ways to comfort, nurture, distract, and resolve your issues without using food. Anxiety, loneliness, boredom, and anger are emotions we all experience throughout life. Each has its own trigger, and each has its own appeasement. Food won't fix any of these feelings. It may comfort for the short term, distract from the pain, or even numb you into a food hangover. But food won't solve the problem. If anything, eating for an emotional hunger will only make you feel worse in the long run. You'll ultimately have to deal with the source of the emotion, as well as the discomfort of overeating.

In most cultures, food is used to celebrate, to comfort, and to nurture family and friends. It's no wonder that we learn to connect emotions and eating. When you add dieting to the mix, however, it wreaks emotional havoc: studies show that dieters have an increased risk of using food to cope with their emotions (Péneau et al. 2013). This is another important reason to reject dieting and practice the tools of Intuitive Eating!

It might be hard to believe, but each act of eating in your life has served you in some way, but some acts have caused you emotional distress and physical discomfort. On a basic level, eating offers nourishment, pleasure, and sometimes comfort. For some people, eating becomes a way of managing or escaping emotions—numbing your feelings. This can range from choosing not to eat (food restriction) to emotional overeating.

This chapter focuses on overeating, but any eating behavior that you engage in for the purpose of escaping emotions is a way of using food to cope. There doesn't necessarily need to be drama and angst involved. Some people use food in this way to deal with a prolonged stressful event, such as a divorce or taking care of a dying relative, but many others are trying to cope with the ordinary and minor irritations of life, like boredom.

The manner in which you were raised can impact your ability to effectively cope with life's ups and downs. If your parents or caregivers helped you develop positive coping skills, such as the ability to speak up, to show emotions, and to receive comfort from others, life's challenges (and irritations) can more easily be met. On the other hand, if your parents were emotionally distant, abusive, or neglectful, or simply unable to cope with problems themselves, you may find yourself turning to destructive coping mechanisms, because you learned no other way to manage life's challenges. When you throw dieting into the fray, you may find yourself catapulted into seeking solace in food, regardless of how you were raised.

The activities in this chapter will help you to:

- distinguish between emotional eating and non-attuned eating as a result of insufficient self-care;

- evaluate the pros and cons of emotional eating;

- identify underlying feelings and how these feelings may trigger the need to cope by using food;

- identify what you are feeling and what you *really* need in those times when you want to continue eating even though you aren't hungry and your body doesn't need any nourishment;

- strengthen your coping mechanisms for dealing with your feelings; and

- learn to prepare for and rehearse stressful events.

Detecting Your Vulnerability to Eating Problems: It Might Not Be Emotions!

Many people believe that they are compulsive overeaters or binge eaters because they watch themselves eat excessively. In fact, many of these people are misdiagnosing themselves. Before you can explore the emotional connections you may have with eating, it's first imperative to determine whether your non-attuned eating is actually based on difficulties you are having handling emotions. Or, rather, is it a consequence of lacking self-care or of the deprivation you feel from a lingering diet mentality?

Self-Care: Reevaluating the Basics

If self-care is lacking, it's hard to be attuned and accurately hear the inner cues of hunger and fullness. Under these circumstances, food can become more rewarding. Review the Self-Care Assessment you completed in chapter 2 and reflect on how you are doing. Then proceed with the rest of this section, which provides a more in-depth look at several key components of self-care: sleep, life balance, nourishment, and stress.

SLEEP

The National Sleep Foundation's (http://www.sleepfoundation.org) research has shown that the optimal amount of sleep for a teenager is eight to ten hours per night; and for an adult, seven to nine hours. If you are not consistently getting adequate sleep, it's likely that you're walking around feeling lethargic, with low energy.

Many people who are sleep deprived believe that their lack of energy can be corrected by eating more. And while it's true that digested food releases physical energy from calories to keep the body functioning and to perform daily tasks, extra food doesn't compensate for a lack of sleep. Eating doesn't wake you up—in fact, it can actually make you feel more sluggish and drowsy.

What can you do to increase the hours and quality of sleep you get per night?

- Turn off all electronic devices early in the evening. Exposure to the light from computer, phone, and television screens is known to stimulate the brain and keep you awake. (You may want to consider changing to "night shift" to reduce the impact of the light on your mobile phone.)

- Set the intention to go to bed at approximately the same time each night and to get up at the same time every morning—even on weekends.

- Exercise during the day to promote better sleep.

- Keep your bedroom cool.

- Avoid caffeine after the morning hours. Caffeine can stay in your system for up to ten hours.

- Reduce alcohol intake. Although alcohol is a depressant, which initially makes you feel relaxed and sleepy, research shows that it actually disrupts your sleep and interferes with your body's sleep regulation (Paddock 2014).

List which of these changes you could make to improve your sleep patterns:

_____

_____

_____

LIFE BALANCE

Sometimes it feels like an impossible task to keep all the balls rolling in your life. Often this is a problem of abundance. There may be many aspects of your life that appeal to you, but you may not have the time for them all. Or it could be an abundance of life's problems. In either case, make it an important goal to be realistic about how much time you can spend in any one area of your life.

Think about the balance among the following aspects of your life: work, play, family, movement, rest, and relationships. Where do you think your life might be out of balance (if at all)?

_____

What can you do to reduce the time you spend on certain areas to provide more opportunities for other aspects of your life, which are currently taking the back seat? (For ideas, you can review the Self-Care Assessment in chapter 2.)

_____

_____

_____

_____

NOURISHMENT

When you eat consistently and adequately, you'll avoid entering a state of primal hunger, which often results in overeating when your brain senses semi-starvation. If you're struggling with this, it is important to review the practices in chapter 2, Honor Your Hunger.

- Do you eat at least three meals and two snacks a day, without going too long between eating? Yes _____ No _____

- Does each of your meals have a balance of protein, carbohydrates, and fat? Yes _____ No _____

- Have you recently increased your amount of physical activity? Yes _____ No _____

- Did you start a new medication, which may have increased your hunger?
  Yes _____ No _____

- Have you changed your pattern of eating? That is, have you started eating lighter meals or having a snack instead of a meal? Yes _____ No _____

Reflect on your responses:

_____

_____

_____

_____

STRESS

Many aspects of life can cause stress—work or school deadlines, moving, separation or divorce, a health crisis for yourself or a family member, or the death of someone close—and stress can have a serious impact on your eating and your health. List some of the stressors in your life:

_____

_____

_____

_____

Consider ways in which you might be able to manage your stress. There are many ways to do this, including getting emotional support from a friend (or a professional), getting physical help (especially in moving), and practicing techniques to overcome procrastinating habits.

_____

_____

_____

_____

The previous exercises helped you identify some factors that may be the source of your overeating. Looking at your life fully and finding the problems that may be affecting your eating—and their solutions—is essential for moving forward in your quest to attune to your body's signals of hunger, fullness, and satisfaction in eating. Without this examination of your life, you may be making the wrong assumption that your eating is purely emotionally based.

Evaluating Your Deprivation Quotient: Stealth Deprivation

Although you have committed to rejecting the diet mentality and making peace with food, you may not be fully healed, which means you may be suffering from what we call *stealth deprivation*. When you are stealth deprived, the habits and patterns of the diet mentality are still rooted in the back of your mind, even though you have tried to eradicate them. The following questions will explore this possibility.

Have you made complete peace with food?

- Do you really believe that all foods are emotionally equivalent? Yes _____ No _____

- Are you able to think about foods without labeling them as good or bad? Yes _____ No _____

- Are you able to eat foods that you truly enjoy at any time, without putting special conditions on them? For example, you don't consider them a treat that should be enjoyed only when you are on vacation or at a wedding. Yes _____ No _____

Do you have food security?

- Do you buy food often enough, so you have a variety of choices and a plentiful amount of food at home? Yes _____ No _____

- Do you have free access to food, rather than it being controlled by someone else, like a family member? Yes _____ No _____

Are any other factors affecting you?

- At social gatherings, have you stopped eating according to the expectations of others rather than eating what you really want? Yes _____ No _____

- Have you stopped eating with judgmental people in your life, who inhibit your food choices? Yes _____ No _____

If you answered no to any of these questions, you may still be living with self-imposed food restriction. Feeling deprived of food (either in the variety or in the amount of food) puts you at risk for overeating, and overeating, of course, often initiates a vicious cycle: food restriction as compensation, rebounding in more overeating, and so forth.

If you are still struggling with the automatic thought that some foods are good or bad, remember that this is a cognitive distortion that has been reinforced by years of diet mentality and by our culture. Use the skills you practiced in chapter 3 (on making peace with food) and in chapter 4 (on challenging the food police) to replace this thought with one that helps you to extinguish this old belief and to replace it with the Intuitive Eating premise that all foods are equal and allowed.

What do you need to do to repair or practice working on these issues?

_____

_____

_____

_____

If you have discovered that some of your disconnected eating is associated with issues of self-care or deprivation from a lingering dieting mentality, there is more work to be done in these areas. Remember, it takes patience and practice. It is best to address these issues before trying to tackle any problems you have with emotional eating. It's much easier to navigate the ups and downs in life when your self-care is in place and the dieting mentality is behind you. The rest of this chapter explores emotional eating and ways to practice new skills for healthier coping mechanisms.

Emotional Reasons for Overeating

It is important to remember that eating does not occur in a void. Much of the time, food has emotional associations. We often forget how deeply food is tied to the need for comfort and safety. This all begins at birth. Soon after a baby is born, he or she is offered milk. That first taste of milk may set the stage for associating pleasure and comfort with a stressful situation. This association deepens when food is offered to soothe aches, celebrate events, and show love—when food becomes a comfort, a reward, and a reliable friend.

Emotional eating covers a wide spectrum of emotions. It can be as positive as pleasure when eating a slice of wedding cake or as destructive as eating to numb difficult feelings or even to punish yourself as a result of negative self-talk.

Evaluating the Pros and Cons of Emotional Eating

It is important to acknowledge how emotional eating has served you. This is the first step toward healing the negative feelings you have about yourself in relation to eating. If you appreciate that you were actually trying to take care of yourself by using or restricting food, when you knew no other way, it will help you to mourn the loss of the behavior as you give it up. And at the same time, it will help you to develop a sense of compassion for your struggle.

Let's begin by exploring how you might have used eating as a coping mechanism. Make a list of recent times when you ate too much or too little or when you ate for any reason disconnected from hunger.

_____

_____

_____

_____

_____

The pros of emotional eating. List the possible ways in which emotional eating has benefitted you, such as offering you comfort, distraction, or a respite from feelings.

_____

_____

_____

_____

_____

The cons of emotional eating. List the ways in which emotional eating has negatively affected your life, such as isolation, physical discomfort, and numbing of positive feelings. (Be sure to approach this list with a nonjudgmental viewpoint. Most people think they've done something wrong when they've used or restricted food to cope with their feelings. Actually, they've only done the best that they could at the time. They've simply grasped for the most accessible coping mechanism they could find—food.)

_____

_____

_____

_____

_____

Do the cons of your eating outweigh the pros? If so, discuss how this is.

_____

_____

_____

_____

If your cons have outweighed your pros, you may be ready to learn to let go of your emotional eating and to find the peace and freedom that comes as you heal.

Identify Emotional Triggers

There are many emotional triggers for eating, and it's likely that most people eat emotionally from time to time:

- anxiety—using food to calm yourself

- boredom—eating as something to do

- bribery—"finish your homework, and you can have a treat"

- celebration—food accompanies most events

- emptiness—eating from a lack of spiritual meaning

- excitement—using food as something fun

- feeling lonely or unloved—using food as a friend

- frustration, anger, rage—eating as a release

- loosening the reins—eating as an outlet from a self-imposed militaristic or perfectionist life

- mild depression—carbohydrates can increase serotonin—the "feel better" neurotransmitter

- self-soothing when upset—eating as a comforting or consoling activity

- procrastination—"I'll do that task after I eat something"

- reward—"I just closed that deal—now I deserve that big piece of chocolate cake"

- stress—food for relief

It is also possible that feelings of *rebellion* can trigger overeating or your food choices. This can happen as a result of reacting to someone in your life. In chapter 4, Challenge the Food Police, you learned that when approached by someone acting like a critical parent, it is common for you to respond like a rebellious child.

List any triggers of emotional eating for you:

_____

_____

_____

_____

_____

Describe some examples of when and how these emotional triggers acted on you:

_____

_____

_____

_____

_____

Become Aware of Your Range of Feelings

Many people are accustomed to avoiding feelings or denying that they have them. To explore the range of the feelings you have, examine the table below, which lists seven core emotions, along with their subsets. These can all be affecting your eating.

Fearful	Angry	Sad	Joyful	Disgusted	Surprised	Ashamed
edgy	exasperated	dejected	amused	appalled	amazed	disgraced
frightened	hostile	gloomy	delighted	contempt	astonished	embarrassed
nervous	irritable	grieved	gratified	disdain	dumbfounded	guilty
scared	outraged	hopeless	happy	indignation	flabbergasted	humiliated
wary	resentful	lonely	satisfied	repulsed	shocked	mortified
worried	vengeful	sorrow	silly	revolted	startled	remorseful

Recall that every emotion has a physical sensation; knowing this is a component of interoceptive awareness. For each of the emotions in the table above, imagine the last time you felt that emotion and reflect upon where in your body you experienced a physical sensation. Part of getting to know your emotional feelings is familiarizing yourself with how these feelings are experienced in your body. The exercise that follows is designed to help increase your awareness of the physical sensations that arise from your emotions. Recalling the emotions from the table above, the next time you are experiencing a strong emotional feeling, write it in one of the spaces in the left-hand column. Pay attention to where it is located in your body, and place an X in the appropriate column or columns to the right. For the last three columns on the right, reflect on the overall body experience—was it pleasant, unpleasant, or neutral? Repeat this exercise for one or two other top emotions, when you experience them. Getting familiar with how emotions feel physically in your body can be the first step in learning to tolerate your feelings.

Getting to Know Your Body—The Physical Sensations of Emotions

Emotion	Head			Chest			Abdomen		Limbs		Overall		
	Eyes	Mouth	Neck	Shoulders	Heart	Lungs	Stomach	Bladder	Legs	Arms	Pleasant	Unpleasant	Neutral

The preceding exercise can be copied or downloaded from the book's website for future use, so you can do it again and again, to help you become more adept at body awareness. Use the following worksheet to assess ways in which you cope with your feelings and how you feel about your life. Put a check by the statements that apply to you. The more checkmarks on this page, the more likely you're using food to cope with your life.

	Coping with Feelings
	1. I eat when I am frustrated, stressed, or upset with myself.
	2. I find myself eating to avoid dealing with problems.
	3. I feel like I have no control over my life.
	4. When a problem arises, it's hard for me to make a plan and follow through with it.
	5. I have trouble saying no when I need to.
	6. My family doesn't support me when I have problems.
	7. I don't like to burden my friends with my problems.
	8. I have difficulty talking about my feelings.
	9. I tend to be impulsive.
	10. I worry about what people think of me.
	11. I feel the need to make others happy.
	12. I don't feel secure in my life.
	13. I have trouble dealing with stressful situations.
	14. I feel out of control with my eating when I feel overwhelmed or stressed out.
	15. I don't trust myself around food.
	16. I often feel hopeless.
	17. I tend to be a people pleaser.
	18. It's hard for me to stop eating when I'm full.
	19. My life seems out of control.
	20. I eat what I really want (such as candy) when no one is around.

Adapted with permission from Ozier et al. 2007; © 2017 Evelyn Tribole / New Harbinger Publications.

Reflection

Review your responses—as a whole, what trend or trends do your responses reflect?

_____

_____

_____

_____

_____

In the next section, you will learn and practice new ways to cope with your emotions, which will help you create a healthier relationship with food.

Healing Emotional Eating

There are three main paths to learning to cope with your feelings without using food:

- Self-Care, Nurturance, and Compassion

- Learning to Sit with Your Feelings

- Helpful Distraction

Self-Care, Nurturance, and Compassion

Self-care, nurturance, and compassion are fundamental to being able to cope with your emotions without using food—they must be established before moving on. They require a belief that not only do you have emotional needs but also that your needs are important and that you have a right to have them met. Without this belief, and without cultivating self-care, nurturance, and compassion, you are likely to continue or return to using food—your original source of comfort and nurturance.

There are many basic human needs that people often deny, but they are essential for self-care:

- enough sleep and rest

- sensual pleasure

- expression of feelings, in order to be heard, understood, and accepted

- intellectual and creative stimulation

- comfort and warmth

Do you often take care of others' needs while negating yours? How does that make you feel—perhaps frustrated, resentful, or exhausted?

_____

_____

_____

_____

Self-nurturance goes beyond the basics of self-care. It's being *extra* nice to yourself. How often (seldom, occasionally, or regularly) do you allow time for experiences that provide self-nurturance, such as the following?

_____

- asking for hugs

- playing with pets

- listening to some soothing or enjoyable music

- reading a book for pleasure

- taking a walk in nature

- looking at a sunset

- buying yourself flowers or another small gift

- getting a massage

- bubble baths, sauna, or steam

- meditating

List your nurturing activities. Be sure to include a couple that don't require money.

_____

_____

_____

_____

Do you crave more nurturance in your life? Think about your typical day, as well as your life in general. Is there time in your life for nurturing activities, or are you overscheduled? List some experiences that you would find nurturing that you don't do now but would like to do.

_____

_____

_____

_____

Having compassion for yourself in this journey is essential. In chapter 4, Challenge the Food Police, we discussed how Intuitive Eating is best thought of as a spiral of healing, with the motto "Come from a place of curiosity, not judgment!" The image of spiral movement reminds you that you should not expect progress to move in a straight line. You will sometimes experience a return to earlier types of behavior, but you should not consider these to be setbacks. When your forward progress loops around into one of these old patterns, look at that movement with curiosity. Use these loops—with their returns to old behavior—to reexamine your beliefs and self-talk and to look again at what you need for self-care. Having an outlook of self-compassion is an essential part of this path to healing emotional eating. When you practice self-care, feel nurtured in the ways that are unique to your life, and speak to yourself with compassion, you will find that eating may no longer serve as your primary source of nurturance. It will become just a way to meet your hunger needs, while providing you pleasure and satisfaction.

USING YOUR IMAGINATION

Along with the types of self-nurturance listed above, you can create a nurturing experience at any moment by imagining a location where you have felt completely calm. This might be at the beach or hiking on a beautiful mountain path. Maybe you're sitting on your couch, wrapped in a soft blanket and listening to music. Or maybe you're at a theater, watching a play or movie.

As you imagine this, ask yourself the following questions: How are you feeling? Are your tense muscles relaxing? Have your racing thoughts slowed down?

_____

_____

_____

Practice imagining yourself in this wonderful, peaceful place. Once you are adept at calling up the image and the warm, relaxing feelings, you will be able to employ them whenever you need them—especially in a moment when you're feeling desperate for food but not hungry.

Learning to Sit with Your Feelings

For some people, it can be an overwhelming task to figure out what you're feeling when you aren't hungry, yet you want to eat, or when you are in the middle of a meal and have had enough to satisfy your physical hunger, but you want to eat more of the delicious food. For some people, however, this situation can be a challenge that offers them a window into their inner world.

TAKING A TIME-OUT: WHAT AM I FEELING RIGHT NOW?

One of the keys to becoming an Intuitive Eater is being willing to take the time to try to figure out your emotional triggers, so that eating is connected to hunger and satisfaction rather than your feelings. It's important to pause—to take a *time-out*—to tune in to these feelings. Even if you eventually choose to eat when you're not hungry or to continue to eat when you're full, a five-minute time-out changes a distracted eating experience into one that is mindful.

Do the following exercise when you find that you are not physically hungry but still want to eat. Before you put any food (or any more food) in your mouth, set a timer for five minutes. Find a comfortable position—sitting or lying down—in a quiet place, without distraction. Explore any of the feelings or emotional triggers you are experiencing that might be causing your desire to eat. What are you feeling right now?

_____

_____

_____

_____

WHAT IS IT THAT I REALLY NEED AT THIS MOMENT?

When the timer goes off, take a moment to ponder if you still have the desire to eat. If your answer is yes, ask yourself, *What do I need—at this moment—to deal with my current feelings?* Since your body isn't hungry, you don't need food. Just notice the answer when it arises. Don't judge it or determine that you can't have what you really need. The answer may come as a storyline: *I need my partner to spend more time with me,* or *I need to speak to my best friend more often,* or *I need some quiet time for myself.*

_____

_____

_____

_____

If your answer came as a storyline, think about the need behind it. Perhaps it is the feeling of connection, the feeling of being nurtured, a sense of spaciousness, or a sense of pleasure and enjoyment.

_____

_____

_____

_____

The next question to ask is *How can I fulfill this need and this feeling without turning to food?* There are many possible answers to this question:

- If you need to feel connection, you might speak up and ask for more time with your partner, or you might schedule some time with friends or family.

- If you need nurturing, you might engage in activities that nurture you, such as painting, hiking, a nap, yoga, or writing in your journal.

- If you seek pleasure and entertainment, you might plan to go to a movie, play, or concert.

- If you need some time alone, you might decide to stay home for the evening to watch your favorite television show instead of going out.

What will work for you?

_____

_____

_____

_____

Repeat this time-out practice regularly to explore these two essential questions: *What am I feeling?* and *What do I really need?* This will be one of your most valuable tools.

BUILDING YOUR EMOTIONAL MUSCLES

If your desire to eat continues to be overwhelming, and you choose to eat, feel free to do so, but be sure to do so without judgment. Don't think that choosing to eat after the time-out exercise is a setback. You are still making progress. The time-out exercise itself is a step forward. Your decision to eat after it is part of the learning process. In the past, you went directly to food the moment an uncomfortable feeling emerged. With this practice, you give yourself the opportunity to identify your feelings and allow yourself to live with them, if only for a few moments, rather than using food to immediately push them away.

Remember, it's important to come from a place of curiosity, not judgment. Be curious about your needs and feelings; don't judge your behaviors. Have patience with this process. Any new behavior takes time to develop and set in. If you end up eating to a point of feeling uncomfortable, be gentle with yourself. Just as the emotions will diminish, so will the physical discomfort. Remember that your body will need food when your hunger returns. Honor your hunger and your body, and feed yourself in a way that is satisfying.

As you continue to do these practices, your *emotional muscles* will grow; you will be able to stay with your feelings for longer periods of time, and, eventually, your need to turn to food when you're not hungry will diminish and disappear.

Note: If your feelings are extremely intense and feel unbearable to you, consider contacting a psychotherapist for a consultation, or if you are already in therapy, connect with your therapist or set up an extra appointment. Some psychotherapists or nutrition therapists allow you to contact them via e-mail when you're in distress. They might not always be able to respond immediately to such emails, but sharing your feelings, and knowing a response will be coming, can be comforting.

THE SADNESS OF SAYING ENOUGH

As you continue practicing taking a time-out, you'll become more adept at being able to wait until you are hungry again to have something else to eat—or to stop eating when you're satisfied and comfortably full. But don't be surprised if *sadness* emerges when you choose not to eat at these times. It's common to feel sad when you have to set a limit to any enjoyable experience. If you allow yourself to experience the sadness, it will pass in just a few moments—especially if you remember that you can eat whatever you wish when your hunger reemerges. If you spend time with this feeling of sadness and acknowledge it, it won't hold power over you.

The following practice is designed to help you when you find that you want to continue eating even though you know that you're comfortably full. You may not be triggered to want to eat more by some deep emotion. It just might be that the food is particularly delicious or that you're simply enjoying the time away from your ordinary tasks. It may feel difficult to stop and set a limit to the amount you're eating, but if this practice is done regularly, it will be part of your emotional growth.

As you notice that you're comfortably full, ask the following questions:

Has this been a satisfying meal, both physically and in regard to taste?

_____

Do I wish to feel physically comfortable—not overly full?

_____

Am I feeling sad that the meal is now over and I need to stop?

_____

Now do the following:

1. For a few moments, sit with the feeling of sadness, as well as with the appreciation you have for the delicious meal.

2. Take a few deep breaths.

3. Now remove yourself from the table. Take the plate to the sink, if you're at home. If you're in a restaurant, ask for a doggie bag (if the food is portable and you like leftovers).

4. If you're at home, go into another room and engage in some other activity.

5. Note how soon the feeling of sadness begins to dissipate.

When you do this practice regularly, you will find a deepened level of contentment in your eating and an increase in your self-esteem, knowing that you can tolerate these feelings of sadness while at the same time appreciating your increasing reconnection with your internal Intuitive Eater.

THE "ONE LITTLE THING" APPROACH

One of the most powerful triggers to overeating is the feeling of being overwhelmed and anxious when life's demands seem to multiply exponentially. There are the demands of work or school, e-mails to answer, phone calls to make, papers to file, as well as bills, household chores, and all of the commitments of your personal life. The best coping mechanism when this occurs is to commit to picking just one task to do in the moment, while letting go of the worry about everything else. Pick just one paper to file or one article to read or one phone call to return. When this one task is finished, you can pick the next.

Do this exercise when you're feeling overwhelmed. Do you feel less anxious? Does it reduce your desire to eat in order to push away the anxiety?

_____

_____

_____

_____

By doing these practices regularly, you will find that the activities you choose will give you more fulfillment and physical and mental well-being than the unnecessary food would have provided.

Helpful Distraction

You might find it odd to see the word *distraction* in the context of learning to cope with your feelings without using food. You've seen that learning to nurture yourself is a prerequisite to being able to have the strength and fortitude to manage the difficult feelings you encounter in your life's journey. You've also practiced the skills of sitting with your feelings as you develop your emotional muscles. So why should we ever consider *distraction* as an option? The answer is that we need to be practical and realistic. Sometimes we simply just need a respite from the pain. We need to find a nondestructive activity that can give us an alternative to difficult feelings and that might give us some satisfaction, joy, laughter, or a way to rest. Just as you need to have rest days from physical exercise so your sore muscles can heal, sometimes you may need to have a time-out from your emotions so that your emotional muscles can heal.

There are many activities that can offer distraction when you need it, including

- going to a movie or watching one at home;

- putting on some music and dancing;

- working on a crossword or jigsaw puzzle, or Sudoku;

- reading an absorbing book;

- flipping through the pages in a magazine; and

- playing a game on the computer.

Give yourself permission to *not* be with your feelings and to pick an activity in which to immerse yourself. What activities might you enjoy when you just can't feel anymore?

_____

_____

_____

_____

In this section, you have explored three paths toward healing emotional eating:

- self-care, nurturance, and compassion

- learning to sit with your feelings

- helpful distraction

Remember that food has helped you cope with life's challenges when you knew no other way to cope. By practicing the exercises in this section, you will find that you are developing and strengthening new coping mechanisms, which will free you to put food in its proper place—for nourishment and satisfaction, rather than for dealing with feelings. Remember to be gentle and compassionate with yourself for having developed your previous coping mechanism of using food. It was the best you could do at the time!

Prevention

Up to this point, you have been dealing with triggers to emotional eating. Now, let's explore ways to help lower your risk of emotional eating during vulnerable times, such as potentially stressful social interactions. This will keep you from being caught off guard.

Preparation

Let's say that you are about to attend a stressful event. It might be a family wedding, a party, an office event, or a vacation with friends. You may start to feel the anticipatory anxiety that typically arises when you're with certain people, especially family. In fact, this anxiety may have been the original trigger that caused you to start using food to calm yourself as a child. There are many ways you can proactively prepare for this kind of stressful gathering.

If you will be out of town:

- Consider staying at a hotel, rather than with family, to give you some built-in boundaries and space.

- If you're staying in someone's home, ask if it's okay for you to bring some foods you like. Don't worry about being judged. Many people have allergies or food sensitivities—your host will likely understand. Or you might want to bring some nonperishable foods, such as nuts or dried fruit, which you could keep in your room without asking at all.

- Bring your walking shoes, so that you can take a break from the gathering and go out for a walk.

- Bring a journal (digital or paper), so you can write about your feelings.

- Put a yoga app on your phone or tablet, so that you can experience the calming effects of yoga while you're away.

There are a few additional strategies that will help whether you're away or in town at an event:

- Ask a close friend—or your therapist or nutritionist—if you can contact him or her if you're beginning to feel difficult emotions. You might not even need to speak to the person. Just knowing that you can leave a message or text might be calming enough.

- Find some safe people, wherever you are, who might be able to comfort you.

- Be sure to take moments for regular deep breathing.

- Practice speaking up in order to get your needs met, and practice setting boundaries with people who might make uncomfortable demands upon you.

- Plan an exit strategy, just in case things get too stressful or you simply need some space. For example, you might say that something has come up at work and that you have to leave.

Choose a few potential stressful situations where there may be a risk of emotional eating. List them here:

_____

_____

_____

List the strategies you might use for each of these situations:

_____

_____

_____

_____

Rehearsal and Visualization

When you visualize a future action or behavior that you would like to accomplish, you focus your mental energy on this task. In this act of focusing, you are actually creating stronger neural networks and altering your brain growth. Athletes regularly practice visualizing making that basket or kicking a field goal in order to increase performance. Likewise, this technique can be utilized to work with eating challenges. You can rehearse an upcoming event by visualizing it. For this exercise, try using one of the stressful situations you listed above.

Imagine being in the situation that is causing you to worry. Visualize that it's time for the food to be served. When you have a clear image of this event, answer the following questions:

1. Which emotions and physical sensations might you expect to feel? What challenges might trigger your urge to overeat or restrict? Perhaps a conversation with a family member? Maybe feeling stressed from traveling? Perhaps excessive downtime, without any activities?

_____

_____

_____

2. When you visualize the dining part of the event, what feelings might you experience?

_____

_____

_____

_____

3. If these feelings seem difficult to manage, what strategies might you use to avoid overeating or restricting?

_____

_____

4. What would it feel like to eat excessively or restrict?

_____

_____

_____

5. Now, imagine what it might be like to stay true to your body's signals and eat only for hunger. If you did not push down your feelings with excess food or by restricting, might you be in emotional distress? What could you do to comfort yourself?

_____

_____

_____

6. What positive feelings might arise as a result of your ability to cope with this stressful event without using or restricting food?

_____

_____

_____

_____

You may have eaten emotionally for many years to numb feelings that were difficult to bear. Just as you wouldn't expect to be able to run a marathon if you've been sedentary for a long time, it would be unreasonable for you to expect to be able to readily tolerate difficult feelings in these types of situations right away. Remember, just as you must build physical muscles to become an athlete, you must develop your *emotional muscles* to be able to tolerate feelings.

Wrap-Up

The tendency to eat emotionally could provide you with a strange gift. Any time that you find that you're craving food when you're not hungry (or wanting to restrict eating when your body needs nourishment)—stop for a moment to appreciate that this urge is actually a voice from within. It's letting you know that there is an emotion or a need that requires your attention. Contemplate what this might be and tap into that well of wisdom from within—you will find the appropriate fit for this emotion or need.

By continuing to practice the exercises in this chapter, it will become easier to identify and examine your triggers and your emotions related to eating. You will have a growing toolbox of helpful techniques. With regular practice, you will discover that your life experience expands exponentially, so that food takes its proper place—as a source of nourishment and one of life's simple pleasures.

In the next chapter, you will learn how to honor your body by practicing techniques that reflect appreciation and respect.

CHAPTER 8

Principle Eight
Respect Your Body

Accept your genetic blueprint. Just as a person with a shoe size of eight would not expect to realistically squeeze into a size six, it is equally as futile (and uncomfortable) to have the same expectation with body size. But mostly, respect your body, so you can feel better about who you are. It's hard to reject the diet mentality if you are unrealistic and overly critical about your body shape.

The dictionary definition for *respect* includes words like *honor, regard, admiration, reverence, esteem, politeness, courtesy, civility, deference,* and *dignity.* Sadly, we rarely hear people describe their bodies in this manner. We live in a culture of body bashing and body shame, thanks to the proliferation of crash-diet programs, social media, and abusive television shows bullying people under the guise of health. As if the human body can be sculpted at will and into a different shape or size!

It's all too common for the chronic dieter to have disdain for his or her current body. But it is important to remember that this body is your home for the rest of your life; it can move you from place to place, can comfort a loved one with a hug, and can give pleasure. Often, it can birth a child and can carry and care for that child.

Respecting your body means treating it with dignity and kindness, as well as meeting its basic needs. In this chapter, you will do exercises that will help you learn to

- accept your body's genetic blueprint;

- have gratitude for your body;

- practice respectful behaviors toward your body;

- stop comparing your body to others; and

- alter the language you use when speaking about your body.

You Can't Fool Mother Nature!

Each of us is born with a genetic blueprint that determines our potential height, weight, and health, as well as a myriad of other details, from foot length to eye color. When you are attuned to your hunger and fullness signals and maintain regular movement and activity, you will be able to maintain and preserve the greater potential of your body. We know, however, that environmental factors can influence our ability to reach this potential or can actually destroy it. Starvation in early childhood can permanently affect bone and tooth growth; malnutrition can damage all organs and increase the risk of infection, communicable disease, and even death.

Most cases of starvation and malnutrition are caused by poverty, war, and abuse, but their damaging results can also be brought on by one's attempt to fool Mother Nature. The power of culture can also wreak havoc on logic. In Chinese history, we know that the cultural ideal of women having small feet caused many to allow their daughters' feet to be bound at a young age in order to force the feet to develop into a deformed—but very small—shape, essentially crippling them. In that era, people believed that a woman needed to have small feet in order to have status and marry into the right family. In our modern world, we live with a culturally thin ideal. Whether it comes from images in the media, the fashion and beauty industry, or family pressure, we see the relentless drive to lose weight, to change how the body looks, and to create an image that is impossible to attain or maintain. Combine these cultural issues with the purported health implications of obesity, and you get a perfect storm for body dissatisfaction.

One can lose weight rapidly (and dangerously) through an eating disorder like anorexia, which, if not treated, will cause health consequences similar to those of outright starvation. One can temporarily lose weight through dieting. But as has been described a number of times through this workbook, diets simply don't work. Even worse, dieting promotes weight gain beyond pre-diet weight; this has been demonstrated in children, teens, and adults. And, yet, people continually try to fool Mother Nature, believing that they can achieve and keep their fantasy body.

The first step in respecting your body is to accept that your body is destined to maintain its genetic blueprint. The few who give up on dieting fairly soon after they begin this futile behavior may be fortunate enough to have a resilient body that returns to its initial blueprint. The majority of dieters, however, attempt one diet after another throughout life, risking a slowed metabolism, an increased fat-to-muscle ratio, and a weight that doesn't resemble that which was originally programmed for their body. How often do we hear people say, "I just looked at a picture of myself in my teens [or twenties or even fifties], when I hated my body! I would give anything to have that body back now!"

Stop the madness; stop trying to fool Mother Nature! Surrender to the body you were meant to have. Treat it with love, respect, self-care, healthful living, and joy. The freedom you will achieve as a result will allow you to place your focus on life goals that are truly achievable and maintainable.

Your Life Without Body Negativity

Unfortunately, many worthy, interesting, kind, and beautiful people hold such negative views about their bodies that they fail to see everything else about them that is positive.

What negative views do you hold about your body?

_____

_____

_____

_____

Imagine what your life would be like if you gave up negative views about your body and the notion of attempting to change it. What would the freedom from worries about your body feel like? What new changes could take place in your life?

_____

_____

_____

_____

What feelings emerge as you work toward dropping your negative body image and accepting Mother Nature's blueprint for your body?

_____

_____

_____

Ways to Show Your Body Respect

Even if you are not fully ready to accept your body's genetic blueprint, and even if you don't like your body, you can still cultivate habits that are kind and respectful toward it.

Gratitude

A study on the effects of gratitude on physical and psychological well-being concluded that a conscious focus on blessings may have emotional and interpersonal benefits, especially positive mood (Emmons and McCullough 2003). In another study (Wood et al. 2008), researchers found that gratitude protected people from stress and depression.

For those who have shown little respect for their bodies for many years, the idea of showing gratitude for a body that they deem to be inferior may sound ludicrous. Yet, if gratitude can be approached with an open mind, most people can find something about their body that they appreciate:

- the ability to walk (a benefit that becomes quite apparent after breaking a leg or injuring one's knee!)

- the ability to engage in sports or leisure activities

- the gift of receiving pleasure, whether from massage, sex, or even scratching an itch

- for a woman, the ability to carry and deliver a healthy baby

- the ability to pick up and play with a baby or toddler

What can your body accomplish? Do you feel gratitude for these abilities?

_____

_____

_____

_____

Self-Care

The concept of self-care is a thread that runs through many of the Intuitive Eating principles. You can show respect by routinely caring for your body in simple and straightforward ways:

- regularly showering, washing your face and hair

- brushing and flossing your teeth

- moving your body through pleasurable physical activity

- including some nutritious foods in your daily food intake

- getting enough restorative sleep

If you don't practice some of those basic elements of self-care consistently—or at all—choose one of those that you need to improve on and practice it for a week. After you consistently improve in one area, add another one, until you've adopted or improved on most of them.

How often are you willing to commit to it?

_____

_____

_____

_____

Getting Rid of the Scale

One of the most immediate ways to show respect to your body is to stop weighing yourself. Stepping on the scale has the power to ruin your day—or give you a temporary high, which is quickly deflated. The scale is a meaningless measure of what is truly important—eating foods that are satisfying, honoring your hunger, and consistently stopping when you're comfortably full. The number that appears on the scale may bring you back to the worship of thinness and the delusion that you can actually permanently change your size, with all the fantasies of the life that will magically arrive with a lowered weight. It completely disconnects you from the important and real and meaningful aspects of your life. The following practice can help to release you from the tyranny of weighing yourself.

Begin by visualizing the last time you got on the scale.

1. How did you feel before you stepped on? Were you feeling anxious, hopeful, or filled with dread?

_____

_____

_____

2. After you saw the number, how did it change your mood and how you felt about yourself?

_____

_____

_____

3. Did the number on the scale affect how you ate that day? Did it make you think that you should eat less that day—or perhaps it gave you permission to eat more, because the number was lower than you had expected?

_____

_____

_____

If you feel an urge to get on the scale this week after completing this exercise, continue to go through the steps above in order to become aware of the negative impact that weighing yourself creates. Remember to check in with your thoughts and feelings as you continue this practice. If you do weigh yourself, try answering the following questions afterward.

1. Write about your feelings before and after you choose to weigh yourself.

_____

_____

_____

2. Now consider whether you would choose to continue this experience, remembering any negative feelings which might have arisen.

_____

_____

_____

3. Are you willing to consider throwing away your scale? If not, what's the first step you could make toward weighing yourself less often and, ultimately, not at all?

_____

_____

_____

Many people experience both exhilaration and dread when they contemplate and ultimately follow through with the task of throwing out the scale. This proactive act asserts your commitment to taking your focus off weight and putting it on attunement to the signals from your inner body wisdom. It may feel scary at first, but it will ultimately feel liberating.

Another assertive action you can take is to decline to be weighed at your doctor's office. Unfortunately, many people avoid doctor visits, even when sick, because of their anxiety about being weighed. They fear their doctor's judgment, as well as their own. You have a right to speak up and refuse to get on the scale. There are very few circumstances in which your actual weight can make a difference in a health assessment. Those might include pregnancy, the calculation for certain medications, and congestive heart failure. In those instances, it is helpful to speak with your doctor about your feelings in order to elicit support. Under those circumstances, you can request not to be shown the number on the scale.

Stop Body Checking

Congratulations, if you have made peace with removing the scale from your life! This is the first step in changing negative self-assessment habits. Remember, respecting your body means treating it with loving care, independent of your size or weight. Unfortunately, people often continue checking their bodies in other ways in order to measure if they're "good enough":

Some people, for example, keep a pair of pants in the closet that are pulled out to "measure" if weight has changed. If the pants are tighter, it can engender the same negative feelings that they would experience if they saw the number on the scale go up. You can combat this kind of measuring by wearing different clothes each day, so that you don't create a muscle memory of how any particular pair of pants feels.

Some people check out mirrors in elevators, dressing rooms, and gyms, and just about anywhere else a mirror can be found. This mirror checking only perpetuates the judgment people hold about how they measure up to the illusion of a perfect ideal body. Remember the fun-house mirrors you laughed at when you were a kid? Most mirrors aren't quite that distorted, but they certainly don't give you an accurate view of yourself. Putting that much attention on your appearance only skews your broader sense of your self and the whole spectrum of your attributes.

Throw Out Old Clothes

Another healing experience is to box up the clothes that are associated with dieting and that no longer fit. If you're not ready to throw them out or give them away (especially if they have sentimental value), you can put the box in the back of your closet or in the garage. Later, when you feel ready, you can get rid of them. Since you bought the clothes when you were trying to lose weight, they will likely not fit your normal body size, which is maintained through eating intuitively and healthy activity. Remember, part of your commitment to this process is to rid yourself of the diet mentality. Holding on to these clothes keeps you stuck in the fantasy that comes with every new diet. Letting go of these clothes will be liberating. When you open your closet door, you won't feel that pang of despair that you feel when you see clothes there that you know don't fit.

Wear Comfortable Clothes

The flip side of throwing out your old diet-tainted clothes is to keep, wear, and occasionally buy only clothes that fit well and are flattering. Wearing clothes that are too tight only makes you uncomfortable and doesn't show respect to your body. This goes for underwear as well. Tight underwear may feel as if you're wearing a straightjacket. Tight clothing makes you feel closed in and trapped, and sometimes you can't even take a deep breath.

Evaluate your wardrobe. Are there clothes that need to go? Are there clothes that don't feel flattering? Respect your body by taking this inventory of your closet and taking the actions you need to restore joy in your clothing.

The following exercise you may want to do while standing in front of or in your closet. Write about the clothes in your closet and what actions you need to take.

Begin by packing away any clothing

- that doesn't make you smile when you look at it;

- that you know fit you only when you were at an unreasonably low weight from dieting or illness; and

- that may fit but is either unflattering, stained, or ripped.

After cleaning out your closet, how do you feel?

_____

_____

_____

_____

Buying New Clothes

Now that you have removed your uncomfortable clothing from your closet, it may be time to buy some new clothes. There are some steps that will help make this experience a success:

- Choose a day of shopping when your emotions are either neutral or positive.

- Start by taking some clothes off the rack—some jeans, for example—in a range of sizes.

- In the dressing room, turn your back toward the mirror, so that you're not looking at it.

- Try on one of the pairs of jeans you have chosen.

- Stretch, contort, wiggle, and sit in them.

- If these jeans don't feel comfortable, take them off, without looking at the mirror, and try on another brand or size.

- If—and only if—they feel comfortable, turn and look in the mirror to see if they pass your style test.

- If you find a pair that feels great and passes your style test, then go right up to the register and buy them!

The point is to buy clothes based on how they *feel*. If they fit well, you won't go around tugging at yourself and feeling uncomfortable with something you think looks good but doesn't feel good.

Stop Comparing

A powerful sign of self-esteem is the ability to maintain an autonomous sense of one's self-worth. Appreciate the myriad of values that are truly yours—the gifts with which you were born. Practicing and refining your talents, and acknowledging the work you have already done to learn and grow, all show a sense of self-respect. Comparing yourself to others leads to unnecessary suffering, which engenders feelings of superiority or envy. Rather than comparing, start appreciating your unique qualities that have nothing to do with appearance!

YOUR PERSONAL QUALITIES

List some aspects about yourself that you particularly appreciate. Reflect on traits, characteristics, and values that you possess that have nothing to do with your body or appearance. They could include personal gifts, such as your intelligence or ability to sing or dance; things that you've worked hard to achieve, like your academic or professional career; or other things, like your friendships and family life:

- intelligent

- funny

- compassionate

- a good listener

- a good spouse, parent, or friend

- patient

- a hard worker

- artistic or musical

- loving

- generous

- thoughtful

Without rushing, write down as many qualities as come to you: _____

_____

_____

_____

_____

_____

Many people shy away from appreciating the personal gifts that are truly theirs—the many qualities and attributes that make them unique—and yet they tend to regularly compare themselves with others to see how they measure up. *Did Sarah get a better score on the test or the term paper than I did? At the office, will I get a raise or a promotion before Michael does? Am I being asked out on as many dates as my best friends are? Am I publishing as many research studies or books as my peers?* It goes on and on.

BODY COMPARISON

The problem of comparing yourself to your friends and peers extends to the focus on the body. Who has the best hair, the smoothest skin, the strongest muscles, the longest legs, or the smallest waist? We make these judgments about our bodies by regularly checking out friends, relatives, actors, models, and just about anyone you see on the street. This attention on others is the surest way to remove you from your own special qualities. It also keeps the focus on the external, and pulls you away from your true meaning in life.

Observing another's body also makes an assumption about how that person achieved that body. If one is looking at thinness, there's no way to know if that person has a physical disease that causes weight loss, has an eating disorder, or simply has a hyper-fast metabolism. Concluding that you could achieve that same body precludes these unknowns, as well as the science of your genetic blueprint. All in all, comparing yourself to others is the surest way of making you feel bad about yourself!

The following is designed to help you become aware of your habit of comparison.

1. How often do you check out others' appearance, clothing, size, or anything else external? List some of the people whom you check out.

_____

_____

_____

2. Notice how you feel when you compare yourself to another. Do you feel inferior, sad, or hopeless? Or perhaps you feel superior and even haughty, when you think you look better than another person. What are your typical feelings?

_____

_____

_____

3. Think of a recent time when you found yourself caught in the comparison trap and ultimately felt "less than." Take a moment to remember how you felt—absorb all of the emotions you felt in that moment. Now refer back to your practice on gratitude and the list of your personal values, and contemplate who you are as an individual and what your unique gifts and qualities are. How do your emotions and feelings change after you've shifted your attention back to your own positive qualities?

_____

_____

_____

THE "AND" PRACTICE—TAKING THE FOCUS OFF BODY IDENTIFICATION

This practice acknowledges that you might be feeling truly uncomfortable in your physical body. But rather than staying stuck in this sensation or identity, it's important to remind yourself of some of your other qualities that you value that have nothing to do with appearance.

- Use a neutral, nonjudgmental description of how you are physically feeling in your body. Don't use loaded words like *puffy* or *flabby*, which can impose a moral judgment on you. Instead, use words such as *uncomfortable* or *challenging*, which acknowledge the physical sensations without playing into the hand of societal expectations. For example, *I am having a difficult body day*, or *I feel physically uneasy in my body today*.

- Add *and* to the above description, and then add three things you admire about yourself (refer to your list of personal qualities above, if you need to). For example, *I am having a challenging body day, AND I am a good listener, a great teacher, and a hard worker.*

Now it's your turn. Create a statement that you could say to yourself when you are having a rough time in your body.

_____

_____

_____

ENVY

Envy is a normal human emotion. It arises when you see someone who has something that you perceive you don't have. You believe that if you had it, your life would be much better. It's likely one of the most difficult emotions to bear. Often when people choose to compare themselves with others, they do this in the hope of finding something they can criticize in the other person. This gives them a temporary sense of superiority as they put the other person down, while elevating themselves in comparison. Thus, the feeling of envy is momentarily avoided. Paradoxically, a switch quickly happens, and they begin to focus on some quality that the other person has that they covet. Envy immediately emerges, and it's likely that they feel even worse despair when they conclude that the other person is actually "better" than they are or has more than they do.

For this practice, first focus on your feelings of envy. How often do you feel envy of aspects of others' lives or their bodies? Frequently? Sometimes? Rarely?

_____

When you feel that envy, are you able to sit with it? Or do you try to find a way in which you believe you are better than the other person? Notice how this makes you feel.

_____

_____

_____

_____

How quickly does this sense of being better than the other person shift back to a feeling of not being good enough? Do you then feel a desire to perfect yourself?

_____

_____

_____

Regardless of how you feel, remind yourself that envy is a normal emotion. When you become comfortable accepting this feeling, your desire to act out against it—by putting someone else down in order to bring yourself up—will diminish. You won't get the immediate rush of superior feelings that emerge, but you'll avoid the potential to crash afterward. Again, direct yourself to feelings of gratitude for your own personal gifts and values.

Body Bashing

One of the most disrespectful behaviors in which you can engage is negative body talk or body bashing. It is painful and sad to hear someone tearing down her or his looks, physique, weight, size, or height. People who would never say anything nasty to a child or a friend or acquaintance—even someone who is not close to you—will say horrific things to themselves. (Side note—we have heard some frightening tales of clients who have been degraded, criticized, and judged by their parents, siblings, or partners. These are instances of emotional abuse and need to be addressed with a trauma therapist.)

This practice will help you to recognize, acknowledge, and put a stop to your self-abusive, body-bashing comments.

1. Recognize your critical body thoughts. Pay attention to your self-talk at times when you are likely to examine your body:

   • taking a shower

   _____

   _____

   _____

   • getting dressed

   _____

   _____

   _____

- catching a glimpse of yourself in a mirror

_____

_____

_____

2. Acknowledge how these thoughts make you feel in that moment. Do you feel anxious, shameful, or sad? Would you acknowledge something like, *These thoughts are not helping—and they are making me feel awful about myself?*

_____

_____

_____

3. When you find yourself engaging in body bashing, narrate your surroundings and describe what you see and hear. (You can do this as an inner monologue or speak out loud—whichever is more comfortable for you.) For example, let's say you're walking someplace and catch your reflection in a mirror or in the window of a nearby building, and you start thinking body-bashing thoughts (such as *My legs are so big—I'm disgusting*). When you find yourself doing this, follow these steps:

Stop.

Narrate. Using a neutral, matter-of-fact voice, describe what you see or hear, without editing it. For example, *I see four cars parked on the street. One car is yellow. I hear kids laughing—ugh, I can't stand my legs.*

Notice when the intrusive body-bashing thoughts creep back in. Don't judge; just quietly acknowledge that your mind has strayed and gently continue to narrate what you hear or see. *There go my body-bashing thoughts again; I need to refocus and continue to narrate. I see a silver car. I hear crows squawking.*

In the lines below, practice narrating your surroundings in this manner, and if negative thoughts creep in, acknowledge them and move on.

_____

_____

_____

_____

By using this practice, you are training your mind to focus on things other than your negative thoughts. With time, you will be able to simply stop your critical thoughts, without narrating your surroundings. At this point in your struggle with self-criticism, the narration serves as training wheels, helping your mind refocus. Eventually, you won't need it.

This week, practice this technique for a few minutes a day when you *don't* need it. It will help give you a good foundation, and you will notice that even when there is no emotional charge, the mind tends to wander. You can narrate while you are driving, riding a bus, waiting for an appointment—anything. When you discover that you have become distracted, acknowledge the distraction and gently continue to narrate. The key here is to practice. It doesn't matter how often your mind wanders—the main point of the exercise is learning to notice your wandering thoughts and then refocusing the mind.

Write about this experience with this exercise this week. How often did you need to redirect your thoughts? Did you have any body-bashing thoughts? If you did, how did you feel each time you had one of those negative thoughts? How did you feel when you redirected your thoughts away from that self-criticism and returned to simply narrating the environment?

Negative Body Talk

How often do you find yourself at a party or with a group of friends and the conversation turns to dieting and fat talk? We live in a society that seems obsessed with these discussions, regardless of age, education, or profession. It is pervasive. Unlike polite banter about the weather, these conversations are harmful, because they reinforce weight stigma and body shame. Speaking up in these situations requires bravery. It suggests that you are someone who knows that a person's worth is attached to purpose, kindness to others, and deep values—rather than the size or shape of the person's body. There are many ways to navigate these conversations, depending on your comfort level, ranging from simply not engaging in the talk to asserting yourself or changing the conversation.

- At a minimum, stop (or don't start) talking about people's bodies (including your own), either with judgment or aspiration.

- Speak up and politely challenge others to become aware of their statements and judgments. Many people are not aware of their weight bias, though it is rampant in our culture. And it doesn't occur to many people that speaking with admiration about someone's thinness or weight loss implies a criticism of everyone who does not conform to those social norms. There are a number of ways of doing this:

  - "It hurts me when I hear people degrading themselves based on appearance."

  - "There's so much more to you than your weight—I enjoy hearing your viewpoints about politics, theater, and books. This has nothing to do with your body size."

- Shift the conversation to travel, to a play or movie that you've seen—or actually to anything that does not promote this abusive talk.

  - *Negative body talk*—"I couldn't possibly wear a bathing suit at the beach. I feel so fat!"

  - *Shift the conversation*—"I was near the beach last weekend and saw the most beautiful sunset. If you get a chance to go down there one evening, you won't believe how glorious it is this time of year.

  - *Negative body talk*—"I can't believe how much weight I've gained—no bread or dessert for me tonight."

  - *Shift the conversation*—"Talking about dessert, I had a piece of the most amazing cake at Susie's wedding last weekend. I must find out which bakery they used."

For the following practice, pick a time when you're going to be with several people. Review the possible responses and have some ideas in mind of what you might say if someone starts talking about the latest diet or says something derisive about her body or judgmental about someone else's body. If such a conversation did come up, how did you handle this situation? What did you say to divert the talk or to address it directly? How did you feel during the conversation and afterward?

_____

_____

_____

_____

_____

If others weren't receptive to what you said, how can you strategize to make your point the next time this happens? (This may include accepting that some people might not see your point of view and deciding how you want to invest your emotional energy).

_____

_____

_____

_____

By taking action to stop fat talk and diet talk, you are raising the consciousness of those who don't realize the damage that is being done by their conversation. One person can begin to change the world. Be proud that you are part of that effort!

Formal Assessment of Positive Body Image

Research on body image has historically focused on its negative aspects, such as body shame and dissatisfaction. Fortunately, new studies are exploring the benefits of appreciating your body. Tylka and Wood-Barcalow (2015) developed the Body Appreciation Scale, which defines and validates three key traits of body appreciation:

- Body acceptance, regardless of size or imperfections.

- Body respect and care by engaging in health-promoting behaviors.

- Protecting your body, by resisting the internalization of unrealistically narrow standards of beauty perpetuated by the media.

Body Appreciation Scale

Here is a simplified version of their updated Body Appreciation Scale. It provides a valid measure of one's body appreciation and positive body image. Write yes or a no next to each statement to see how far you have come in respecting your body.

- I respect my body.

- I feel good about my body.

- I feel that my body has at least some good qualities.

- I take a positive attitude toward my body.

- I am attentive to my body's needs.

- I feel love for my body.

- I appreciate the different and unique characteristics of my body.

- My behavior reveals my positive attitude toward my body; for example, I walk holding my head high and smiling.

- I am comfortable in my body.

- I feel like I am beautiful even if I am different from media images of attractive people (e.g., models, actresses/actors).

After assessing these statements, reflect on how many yes responses you made. The more yeses indicate you are making good progress with body appreciation.

If you score only a 1 or 2, remember not to judge yourself. You're on a journey that will help you to have positive thoughts about your body. If you're in a middle range, a 6 or a 7, you've done quite a bit of work. As in other areas of achievement, strive not to look for perfection, simply increased appreciation for your body.

What do you need in order to respect, accept, and love the body you have?

_____

_____

_____

Are you ready to give up the fantasy that you can alter your body to match some unrealistic image? If you are, list the ways that you plan to show yourself that you are sincere in your commitment. There are many ways to do this:

- *I will speak kindly to myself about my body.*

- *I will feed myself regularly and engage in enjoyable physical activities.*

- *I will throw away my scale and give away the old clothes that don't fit my body size.*

If you do not feel ready to let go of the fantasy, contemplate what you might need in order to do so.

_____

_____

_____

Please list as many positive behaviors (including positive self-talk about your body) that you are willing to implement:

_____

_____

_____

_____

It would be helpful to use the statements in the Body Appreciation Scale weekly over the next few months to assess how you are doing. (You can download a handout of the Body Appreciation Scale from the website for this book.) Note how your body appreciation increases over time. Notice whether practicing other exercises in this workbook influences your appreciation of your body.

Wrap-Up

We all come in different sizes and shapes. Our culture accepts foot size and doesn't try to alter it. The same attitude should apply to our bodies. Your path involves acceptance of your size and respect of your body. When you can truly surrender to the reality that no diet, no food restrictions, and no exercise regimen will permanently change your genetically determined size (other than, of course, in a damaging way), you are on your way to truly being kind to your body, treating it with dignity, and, yes, even loving your body. Love it for what it can do for you. Love it by taking good care of it—it has done so much for you. Love it by presenting yourself in ways that appreciate your own personal aesthetic.

The next chapter will examine your relationship with movement and physical activity, while addressing any resistance you may hold toward exercise.

CHAPTER 9

Principle Nine
Exercise: Feel the Difference

Forget militant exercise. Just get active and feel the difference. Shift your focus to how it feels to move your body, rather than the calorie-burning effect of exercise. If you focus on how you feel from working out, such as energized, it can make the difference between rolling out of bed for a brisk morning walk or hitting the snooze alarm. If when you wake up, your only goal is to lose weight, it's usually not a motivating factor in that moment of time.

There is no question that exercise is beneficial for a myriad of health issues from stress reduction to prevention of chronic diseases. The issue for most people is the art of doing it consistently. A big challenge for chronic dieters is choosing the right exercise. If they make their selection based on how many calories they will burn, they might be engaging in activities they don't necessarily find enjoyable.

When your focus is on an unattainable aesthetic, rather than the intrinsic pleasure of movement, you are setting yourself up for disappointment. Worse yet, exercise becomes part of the dieting mentality and drudgery, which leads to burnout. Consequently, when the dieting stops, so does the physical activity, which is understandable—if your primary experience with exercise has been connected with dieting or when you're not eating enough food, you won't learn that exercise can feel good.

Note that we use the term *exercise* interchangeably with *movement* and *physical activity*. The World Health Organization emphasizes that physical activity does not mean only exercise or sports (2010). In fact, these endeavors are subcategories of physical activity, which includes other activities as well, such as playing, gardening, doing household chores, dancing, and recreational activities.

There are two critical components to physical activity and health—less time sitting every day and more time engaging in physical activity itself. A growing body of research shows that sitting too much is not the same thing as exercising too little (Henson et al. 2016; Cheval, Sarrazin, and Pelletier 2014; Craft et al. 2012). Studies show that even if you exercise regularly, it does not protect you from the effects of sitting too much. In this chapter, we explore both of these issues.

In this chapter, you will

- discover physical activities that you enjoy;

- explore the qualities of mindful exercise, while paying attention to the connection with your body;

- identify personal benefits and reasons to exercise;

- discover how to break through exercise barriers; and

- learn how to increase activity by sitting less.

Start By Simply Sitting Less in Your Daily Living

A person can now eat, work, shop, bank, and socialize without having to leave the comfort of their chair.

—Henson et al. 2016

Thanks to technology and urbanization, the average person spends more time sitting than sleeping (Craft et al. 2012). This lifestyle of prolonged sitting is now recognized as a unique health hazard, which increases the risk of chronic diseases, especially heart disease and type 2 diabetes (Henson et al. 2016). When the body sits for long period of time—an hour or more—there is a physiological stasis effect; your metabolic health comes to a standstill.

That's why it is not enough to focus on exercise guidelines (which are still important and will be described later). Studies show that many people who exercise regularly still sit too much and are actually considered to be sedentary. You can be sedentary at work, at school, at home, when travelling, or during leisure time by

- sitting or lying down while watching television or playing video games;

- sitting while driving a car, or while travelling by plane, train, or bus; and

- sitting or lying down to read, study, write, or work at a desk or computer.

Consequently, public health programs are aiming to find ways both to reduce total sitting time and to increase the number of breaks in prolonged sedentary periods—all without the need to break a sweat. Just to be clear, this is not about hopping out of your chair to perform a set of jumping jacks. Rather, it's about simply getting up and breaking the stillness of sitting, which could be as easy as getting up to talk on the phone and continuing the conversation while standing. These types of activities are classified as Non-Exercise Activity Thermogenesis (NEAT) (Cheval, Sarrazin, and Pelletier 2014). They include a wide range of low-intensity behaviors: the ordinary activities of daily living, fidgeting, spontaneous muscle contraction, and maintaining proper posture. Don't underestimate the important role these seemingly mundane activities play in metabolic and cardiovascular health! Even the most incidental tasks of everyday living, like taking out the trash, offer significant health benefits (Rezende et al. 2016).

If you are out of shape, starting with an effort focused on less sitting (or NEAT) is a much less daunting endeavor than beginning with a new fitness regime.

Getting Real: Estimating the Amount of Your Sitting Time

We spend so much time chasing deadlines and running errands that it is easy to perceive that we are living active, rather than sedentary, lifestyles. But for most people, this chase is accomplished while sitting in a car or behind a desk or staring at a smartphone.

First, let's get an idea of what your sitting lifestyle is really like (without judgment, please). The purpose is to provide a better picture of how much time you spend sitting, which will give you a better idea of where it might be feasible to make some easy changes. Select two typical days (one weekday and one day on the weekend). On the following chart, track the hours you spend sitting on those days, and in the right-hand column, note the longest *uninterrupted* period of time spent sitting. If you sat continuously to watch a three-hour movie, you would write down "three hours"—but if you got up to go to the kitchen halfway through the movie, your entry would be "one and a half hours."

Your Sitting Time

	Total Hours in the Day		Hours Spent
Sedentary Pursuits	*Weekday*	*Weekend*	*Prolonged Sitting (uninterrupted, not getting up)*
Driving or sitting in a car, plane, or train.			
Sitting at a desk.			
Watching television or movies.			
Surfing the Internet or engaged in social media, such as Facebook.			
Playing video games.			
Reading.			
Texting, talking, or engaged in social media on your phone.			
Simply relaxing or lounging.			
Total Hours			

Exploring How to Sit Less and Interrupt Prolonged Sitting

After you complete your estimated time spent sitting during the weekdays and weekends, answer the following questions.

How many hours do you spend sitting or lying down during

weekdays _____

weekends _____

What was your longest bout of uninterrupted sitting, and is this typical for you?

_____

_____

Below is a list of ways to interrupt sitting. Read through them and place a checkmark next to those that you would be willing to incorporate into your everyday living.

General Tips

☐ Break up any prolonged sitting with stretching, getting up, turning, or bending.

☐ Take advantage of smartphones and electronic apps to prompt you to get up after forty-five to sixty minutes of prolonged sitting.

☐ Find different ways to sit that engage an active posture, such as perching on a balance ball or a bar stool.

At Home

☐ Set an alarm or preset the timer on your phone to go off every hour to remind you to get up and move in some way: take a stretch break, get the mail, put stray items away, do the laundry, or take out the trash.

☐ Walk around, rather than sitting, when talking on your phone.

☐ Take stand-up breaks while sitting and reading.

☐ Change your reading location, such as from indoors to outdoors, once an hour.

In Your Office or at Your Desk

☐ Take your lunch break away from your desk.

- ☐ Stand while you read at work.

- ☐ Walk around or stand when talking on the phone, perhaps using a headset if that makes it easier or allows for more movement.

- ☐ At meetings, stand rather than sit at a conference table.

- ☐ For small meetings with one or two people, schedule or suggest a walk-and-talk meeting.

- ☐ Move your trash can away from your desk, so you have to get up to use it.

- ☐ Set an alarm on your computer to remind you to stand up and move more often.

- ☐ Consider getting an adjustable standing desk that will allow you to work at different heights from sitting to standing.

Transportation

- ☐ On an airplane, get up and take a stretch break every hour or walk up and down the aisle.

- ☐ On a train or bus, get off one stop earlier than your destination, if practical.

- ☐ In a taxi or car service, such as Uber, get off one block before your destination.

The Pursuit of Pleasurable Activities

A growing body of research shows that deriving pleasure from physical activities may be one of the most important factors for sustaining consistent exercise, rather than focusing on the classic fitness prescriptions of frequency, intensity, and duration (Parfitt, Evans, and Eston 2012; Ekkekakis, Parfitt, and Petruzzello 2012; Petruzzello 2012; Segar, Eccles, and Richardson 2011). This concept of engaging in activities that you enjoy or that give you increased energy or an improved mood is based on the Hedonic Theory of Motivation. This theory basically says that people will repeat activities that feel good. Conversely, activities that cause pain or discomfort will wane or be avoided. This is welcome research, refuting the popular notion that people need to be bullied into physical activity in the name of health.

All too often, people have been cajoled to disregard the cautionary messages of the body with adages such as *suck it up* or *no pain, no gain*. This can lead to a big disconnect, because it encourages pain and minimizes the messages you are receiving from your body. Just as dieting teaches you to ignore what your body wants and needs, these old patterns of exercise only separate you from the wisdom of your body. Remember, only you can possibly know how your body feels.

Let Your Body Be Your Guide: Mindful Exercise

Paying attention to how your body *feels* during and after movement is an important way to discover enjoyable activities. Mindful exercise places value on paying attention to how your body feels—without judgment, comparison, or competition. It is an activity that fosters attunement, which includes four components (Calogero and Pedrotty 2007):

- It rejuvenates, rather than exhausts or depletes.

- It enhances the mind-body connection.

- It alleviates stress, rather than amplifies stress.

- It provides genuine enjoyment and pleasure.

The more you can tune in to your body's sensations during physical activities (not merely thinking about the sensations, but actually *feeling* them), the more it can help you cultivate interoceptive awareness (your perception of the physical sensations from within your body). During exercise, these sensations can include the intensity and rate of your breathing, speed and strength of your heartbeat, muscle tension and muscle relaxation, and overall perceived effort or exertion. The more you listen to your body, the more it heightens your ability to "hear" it, which will also increase your interoceptive awareness in other areas—like perceiving hunger and fullness. Think of it as a form of cross-training for your mind-body connection—all of which are connected and interdependent.

Exploring How the Pursuit of Enjoyable Activities Would Impact You

1. How would pursuing physical activities for pleasure and enjoyment affect your

   A. desire to be active?

   _____

   _____

   _____

   B. selection of type of activity you engage in, especially if you feel out of shape?

   _____

   _____

   _____

C. selection of the environment where you exercise—with others or alone, in public or private, outdoors or in a gym?

_____

_____

_____

2. How would a pleasant physical activity feel to you, during and after you exercise?

_____

_____

_____

3. How would placing an emphasis on activities that are invigorating, rather than exhausting or depleting, affect your choice and frequency of exercise?

_____

_____

_____

Benefits of and Barriers to Physical Activity

Benefits of Physical Activity

While most people know there are many health benefits gained from exercise, it is such a generalized idea that it may lose its specific relevance to you. In this section, we briefly review the benefits of physical activity in two parts: reducing the risk of diseases and improving life-enhancing qualities.

HEALTH BENEFITS OF PHYSICAL ACTIVITY

Review the following chart of the health benefits of physical activity. In the first section, Reduces Health Risks, put a checkmark in the box next to any diseases and conditions that are in your family history (parents, grandparents, and siblings). In the next section, Improves Quality of Life, circle the benefits that are meaningful to you.

Reduces Health Risks	
☐ Cognitive decline	☐ Insulin resistance
☐ Colon cancer	☐ Lung cancer
☐ Depression	☐ Osteoporosis and bone fractures
☐ Endometrial cancer	☐ Premature death
☐ Heart disease	☐ Stroke
☐ Hypertension	☐ Type 2 diabetes
Improves Quality of Life	
Long-term qualities, which take a while to accrue	*Short-term qualities, which you will notice day-to-day*
Bone density	Strength
Grey matter of brain	Balance
Cognition and memory	Mood
Gut microbiota	Stamina
Satiety cues	Appetite regulation
Lean body mass	Stress tolerance
Cardiovascular circulation	Sleep quality

EXPLORING THE SHORT-TERM LIFE-ENHANCING BENEFITS OF PHYSICAL ACTIVITY

In this section, we will focus on the more noticeable short-term benefits of exercise, the things that generally make you feel good. Using the information from the chart above, answer the following questions.

Describe two short-term benefits of exercise that are appealing to you.

_____

_____

How would selecting an activity based on benefits that you actually *feel*, such as improved energy, mood, strength, or sleep, affect your day-to-day quality of life? For example, consider how feeling more energized after an activity would affect you for the rest of the day (or night).

_____

_____

_____

_____

Barriers to Exercise

Despite the well-known health benefits of physical activity, inactivity is a growing problem globally. According to the World Health Organization (2010), inactivity is the fourth leading cause of death—with approximately 3.2 million deaths each year attributable to insufficient physical activity.

Even when you personally value the benefits of exercise and have a genuine desire to be active, there can be obstacles to overcome—some of which may be based on how you experienced play time or sports growing up. Perhaps you were teased or bullied into exercising, which can create a disdain for any activity. Or there may be present-day challenges, such as a demanding schedule with school, kids, work, or a combination thereof. Understanding your barriers to exercise and creating strategies to overcome them can help you make physical activity a regular part of your life.

EVALUATING BARRIERS TO EXERCISE

Review the questions and check the ones that apply to your situation.

Yes	Questions
Teasing, Punishment, or Pressure	
	1. Was exercise ever used as a punishment (such as being forced to run laps or do push-ups for misbehavior)?
	2. Were you teased for being uncoordinated?
	3. Were you the last to be picked for teams?

	4. Were you ever forced to exercise for weight loss?

Dieting Mentality and Rigid Thinking

	5. Do you use exercise to compensate for eating a particular food, such as dessert?
	6. Do you believe you need to be the right size or weight in order to exercise?
	7. Do you believe that physical activity counts only if you sweat and burn a lot of calories?
	8. Is losing weight the primary purpose of exercising for you?
	9. Do you often exercise only when starting a new diet?
	10. Do you set up on unrealistic goals, only to give up on physical activity?

Time, Schedule, and Weather Challenges

	11. Do you feel like you don't have enough time to exercise?
	12. Does your job require a lot of travel?
	13. Do you have a lot of family obligations, with little free time for yourself?
	14. Does the weather affect your ability to exercise outdoors?

Confidence, Conditions, and Equipment

	15. Do you lack confidence about your ability to be physically active?
	16. Have you had an injury or condition (including age) that keeps you from doing what you used to enjoy doing?
	17. Are you afraid of being injured?
	18. Do you feel too tired to exercise?
	19. Do you feel you don't have any comfortable clothes to wear for activities?

EXPLORING BARRIERS TO EXERCISE

Select the barriers that present the biggest obstacles to physical activity for you. Describe what you could do to overcome each barrier.

First Barrier:

_____

_____

Solution: _____

_____

_____

_____

Second Barrier:

_____

_____

Solution: _____

_____

_____

_____

What do you need in order to make physical activity a nonnegotiable priority in your life? Consider how you are doing in self-care and setting boundaries.

_____

_____

_____

_____

OVERCOMING BARRIERS: IMPORTANCE OF A BODY-POSITIVE ENVIRONMENT

If you do not feel comfortable exploring a new activity or fitness endeavor alone, seeking a qualified personal trainer or a gym that has guided group activities can be helpful. Yet far too many people feel out of place at a gym; they don't feel welcome. Worse yet, some gyms and classes are focused on weight loss rather than enjoyment, strength, and energy.

Fortunately, there is a growing recognition on the importance of body positivity within the fitness industry, evidenced by the Body Positive Fitness Alliance (BPFA). The BPFA requires affiliated members and corporations to be trained in and to comply with their seven pillars of body-positive fitness in order to make physical activity more accessible, approachable, and fun. In addition, it promotes an effective community, with exercise professionals who work within their scope of practice and are focused on full health and body positivity. We think the pillars are revolutionary and suggest that people look for these qualities in a fitness environment or trainer.

The Body Positive Fitness Alliance Seven Pillars[*]

1. *Accessibility.* I choose to provide an environment where anyone from any walk of life can step foot in and move their bodies without worrying about what they look like while doing it.

2. *Approachability.* I choose to eliminate any intimidating elements from this space, which I provide. I understand the difference between intimidating and challenging.

3. *Enjoyment.* I apply the fact that people are motivated when they feel like they belong to a community where they can become their best selves and can have fun!

4. *Community.* I have built a community free of egos and full of heart. I have taught my members that "fit" does not have a look. Anyone who walks in our doors is a member of our family. We celebrate each other's successes, we lift each other up when down, and we don't stand for judgment.

5. *Scope of Practice.* I agree that being a fitness professional does not necessarily make one a nutrition professional, a mental health professional or a general health advisor. I refer my clients to appropriate care when their needs are outside of my scope of practice. I can identify and I value evidence-based science. Studied and proven methods drive my practice.

---

[*] Reprinted with permission from the Body Positive Fitness Alliance.

6. *Full Health.* I live in the belief that health is equal parts mental, physical and emotional. Balance is the key to health and one third cannot thrive if another third is suffering.

7. *Body Positivity.* I believe in praise and celebration of what one can do and not what one looks like. I understand the damage which is done to individuals when they are encouraged to take up less space. I empathize with the fact that individuals are unique in shape and size, and one's shape or size does not necessarily indicate their strength, endurance, and overall fitness and health. I understand that happiness does not rely on smallness and fitness does not have a "look."

Discover Physical Activities You Enjoy

In this section you will explore physical activities to try, learn the optimal frequency and duration of exercise, and monitor how your body feels, with the emphasis on enjoyment, of course!

Getting Started

To help you get started with making physical activity an enjoyable part of your life, consider these factors.

1. What are your preferences?

    ☐ Exercising alone or   ☐ with a group of people

    ☐ Exercising indoors versus   ☐ outdoors

2. What is your current fitness level? _____

3. Considering your current fitness level, what would be the most pleasurable type of activities to explore?

    _____

    _____

4. How do you want to feel after physical activity? Perhaps calm or perhaps energized?

    _____

    _____

PHYSICAL ACTIVITIES WORKSHEET

Review this list of physical activities. The five middle columns indicate different aspects of the activities—whether the activity is typically practiced as a game, whether it is a solo or group exercise (or both), and whether it's done indoors or outdoors (or both). In the right-hand column, rate your interest in exploring each exercise from 0 to 10, with 0 being not interested and 10 being very interested.

Activity	Game	Solo	Group	Indoor	Outdoor	Interest (0–10)
Badminton	x		x	x	x	
Basketball	x		x	x	x	
Cycling		x	x	x	x	
Body surfing		x	x		x	
Boogie boarding		x	x		x	
Cross-country skiing		x	x		x	
Dancing				x		
Ballet		x	x	x		
Ballroom			x	x		
Club			x	x		
Hip-hop			x	x		
Jazz			x	x		
Pole			x	x		
YouTube Videos		x		x		
Zumba			x	x		
Dodgeball	x		x		x	
Flag football	x		x		x	
Gardening		x			x	
Geocaching	x				x	

Activity	Game	Solo	Group	Indoor	Outdoor	Interest (0–10)
Gymnastics				x		
Acrobatics				x		
Aerial hoops or silks				x		
Tumbling				x		
Gyrotonics		x	x	x		
Handball	x		x	x	x	
Hiking		x	x		x	
Hula hooping		x		x	x	
Ice skating		x	x	x	x	
Jumping rope		x	x	x	x	
Laser tag	x		x	x		
Kayaking		x	x		x	
Kickboxing			x	x		
Martial arts		x	x	x		
Capoeira		x	x	x		
Karate		x	x	x		
Kung fu		x	x	x		
Jujitsu		x	x	x		
Self-defense		x	x	x		
Tae kwon do		x	x	x		
Tai chi		x	x	x		
Paintballing	x		x		x	
Pilates		x	x	x		
Ping-pong	x		x	x	x	
Playing with your dog		x		x	x	

Activity	Game	Solo	Group	Indoor	Outdoor	Interest (0–10)
Playing with kids	x		x	x	x	
Dodgeball	x		x		x	
Hide-and-seek	x		x	x	x	
Hop scotch	x		x		x	
Tag	x		x		x	
Rocking Climbing		x	x	x	x	
Roller skating or roller blading		x	x	x	x	
Running		x	x	x	x	
Sailing		x	x		x	
Skateboarding		x	x	x	x	
Skiing		x	x		x	
Snowboarding		x	x		x	
Soccer	x		x		x	
Stand-up paddleboard		x	x		x	
Surfing		x	x		x	
Swimming		x	x	x	x	
Tennis	x		x		x	
Trampoline		x	x	x	x	
Video Games	x	x	x	x		
Dance Dance Revolution	x	x	x	x		
Wii Fit	x	x	x	x		
Wii Tennis	x	x	x	x		
Just Dance	x	x	x	x		
Other	x					

Activity	Game	Solo	Group	Indoor	Outdoor	Interest (0–10)
Volleyball	x		x	x	x	
Wakeboarding		x	x		x	
Walking		x	x	x	x	
Weight lifting		x	x	x		
Body pump (weights lifted to music, led by teacher)			x	x		
Circuit weights		x	x	x		
Free weights		x	x	x		
Yoga		x	x	x	x	

EXPLORING PHYSICAL ACTIVITIES

1. List the activities that you gave a rating of 7 or higher for your interest in exploring. Then circle the top three activities that you would like to try. (Note that if none of the activities was appealing enough to get a rating of 7 or above, list some activities that you might tolerate.)

2. What do you need in order to get started? Consider your schedule, comfortable clothing, comfortable shoes, equipment, and a check-up from your doctor.

_____

_____

_____

_____

_____

3. What do you need in order to keep your expectations realistic, especially if you are not fit or if you are trying a new activity, especially one that requires practice to develop the new skills?

_____

_____

_____

_____

_____

How Much Activity and How Often?

Doing some physical activity is better than doing none.

—World Health Organization

In this section, we will explore how much activity to strive for in a week, but as you read, it is important that you keep in mind the World Health Organization's advice: any activity is better than none. When it comes to accruing the health benefits of physical activity, even just short bouts of ten minutes will benefit your cardiovascular health (World Health Organization 2010). Please don't use the recommended exercise targets discussed below to beat yourself up if you currently don't meet the guidelines. It is important to start with where you are at and what is comfortable for you.

HOW MANY MINUTES PER WEEK?

Both the WHO and the Physical Activity Guidelines for Americans recommend the following targets for adults aged eighteen to sixty-four years.

- Aim for seventy-five to 150 minutes of physical activity per week, depending on whether the intensity of the activity is moderate or vigorous (see the next section for details).

- Be sure to include at least two muscle-strengthening activities a week as part of your total time spent in physical activity. (Examples of these types of activities include some types of yoga and lifting weights.)

If you are sixty-five years old or older, the guidelines are the same as above, with an added recommendation for those who have poor mobility: engage in activities that enhance balance and prevent falls at least three days per week.

EFFORT OR INTENSITY

Generally, *intensity* refers to how much effort you put forth in an activity, which can vary from person to person. One way to gauge this effort is using an exertion scale of 0 to 10, where sitting is 0 and the greatest effort possible is 10.

Moderate-intensity activity requires a medium level of effort, about a 5 or 6 on the exertion scale. This effort produces a noticeable increase in your breathing rate and heart rate. Examples of these types of activities include general gardening and walking. Aim for 150 minutes of these types of activities.

Vigorous activity is about a 7 or 8 on this scale, produces a large increase in your breathing and heart rate, and often causes sweating. Examples include tennis, jogging, and hiking on hilly terrain. If you engage in these types of activities, aim for at least seventy-five minutes throughout the week.

A general rule of thumb is that two minutes of moderate-intensity activity counts the same as one minute of vigorous-intensity activity (USDHHS 2008), so thirty minutes of moderate-intensity activity is roughly the same as fifteen minutes of vigorous activity.

PHYSICAL ACTIVITY PLANNING GUIDE

When you start to explore what getting seventy-five to 150 minutes of exercise in a week looks like, it can seem surprisingly manageable. Consider your regular obligations, and use the weekly planning grid below to indicate when and how much activity is realistic for you.

	Target minutes per week	Monday	Tuesday	Wednesday	Thursday	Friday	Saturday	Sunday
Example: Moderate	150		10 minutes walking	10 minutes walking	10 minutes walking		60 minutes yoga class	60 minutes gardening
Example: Vigorous	75	20 minutes jogging		20 minutes brisk walking		20 minutes hiking		15 minutes weights
Week 1								
Week 2								
Week 3								
Week 4								

MONITORING HOW YOU FEEL

It's important to pay attention to how you feel during and after your activity—this will help you prevent injuries, while helping you focus on the sensation of pleasantness during activity and the accruing benefits of movement (such as improved mood and alertness). The following journal is a useful tool to monitor these factors. In the columns on the left, record the date, your activity, and its duration. In the central columns, note how you feel during and after the activity. During your activity, pay attention to the intensity of your breathing, the sensations of your muscles (such as relaxed, tense, or sore), and your overall perceived effort of exertion—then reflect on whether the activity felt pleasant, unpleasant, or neutral. After the exercise, reflect on the less directly physical effects of your activity—did it improve your alertness, mood, or stress levels? Some of these effects you might feel immediately, some later, and these effects may last a long time or be brief. In the right-hand column, make any other comments you would like about the activity.

Activity Journal: Embodied Physical Activity

Date	Activity	Duration (minutes)	How Did You Feel...?						Comments
			During Activity?			After Activity?			
			Pleasant	Unpleasant	Neutral	Alertness	Mood	Stress	

REFLECTION OF ACTIVITY JOURNAL

After you complete a few days of this journal, review it and answer the following questions.

During your activity, how does your perceived effort and the intensity of your breathing affect the pleasantness of your overall experience?

_____

_____

_____

What is the difference between the sensation of feeling invigorated versus feeling exhausted and depleted from an activity?

_____

_____

_____

If your activity felt unpleasant, what could you do to improve your enjoyment? Consider the intensity of your effort, your expectations, and whether you were competitive with yourself or others. Also consider other factors, such as getting enough sleep the night before, how frequently you engage in the activity, and the environment in which your activity took place.

_____

_____

_____

After your activity, what trends did you notice about your overall mood, alertness, and stress level?

_____

_____

Did you notice any other benefits, such as being more eager to take on the day or any improved quality of your sleep?

_____

_____

In the beginning, you might not notice any trends of improved overall well-being. Keep in mind that it takes about twelve weeks to get a physiological effect from moving your body consistently.

EXERCISING TOO MUCH

We have spent most of this chapter on how to overcome too little physical activity, but it's important to recognize if you have crossed over the line into an unhealthy pursuit of compulsive exercise, which could also be a sign of an eating disorder. The table below lists some warning signs to consider. Check yes to the statements that apply to you.

Yes	Warning Signs
	You continue to work out even when you are sick.
	You feel guilty if you skip a day of exercise.
	You decline activities with friends, such as biking or going for a walk, because it seems like a waste of time (that is, you think it isn't vigorous enough to count as exercise).
	You increase the amount of your exercise if you think that you ate too much food or high-calorie foods.
	You feel restless or irritable if you take a day off or try to cut down your exercise.
	You exercise longer than originally intended.
	You lie to friends and family to hide how much time you spend exercising.
	You feel the need to work out longer and longer in order to feel good.
	You decline going out or engaging in other social activities in order to exercise.
	You go through withdrawal when not exercising, such as feeling anxious or depressed.
	You fear that if you stop exercising, you will not be able to return to working out.
	You believe that you have to experience pain in order to gain benefits from exercise (following the mantra no pain, no gain).
	You over-exercise in order to lose weight.

If you find that you are exercising too much, it's important to listen to your body rather than the exercise rules from your mind. This may mean taking some time off from working out and letting your body recover. Keep in mind that you do not get out of shape from missing a few workouts, but you could get sick or injured if you don't take a break. The process of recovering from over-exercise is similar to recovering from the diet mentality. You might need to see an eating disorder specialist.

Wrap-Up

Although it is important to move your body regularly and refrain from prolonged sitting, it is very important to listen to your body. This might mean taking time off if you are sick, injured, or sleep deprived. That's okay—it will keep you healthy and more likely to engage consistently in physical activity, which is important in the big picture of your lifetime.

CHAPTER 10

Principle Ten
Honor Your Health: Gentle Nutrition

Make food choices that honor your health and taste buds while making you feel well. Remember that you don't have to eat a perfect diet to be healthy. You will not suddenly get a nutrient deficiency or gain weight from one snack, one meal, or one day of eating. It's what you eat consistently over time that matters. Progress, not perfection, is what counts.

Getting to the last chapter in this workbook is quite a feat! You've spent many hours challenging old beliefs, assumptions, and fantasies. You've observed your behaviors and thoughts and feelings. You've made peace with food, committed to never going on another diet, learned to figure out what you really feel like eating and what you *really need* when you want to eat but aren't hungry. You've practiced honoring your hunger and feeling your fullness. You've tolerated feelings of sadness when it's time to stop eating a delicious meal and have strengthened your emotional muscles in order to sit with your feelings. You've grown in respect and appreciation for your body and all that it can do for you. You've found a way to bring movement back into your life in a joyous and healthy way. We hope you feel proud of all the work you have done!

Now you're left with one last task—figuring out whether you're ready to face the ever-changing world of nutrition and how to make it work in your life. There was a reason for making Honor Your Health with Gentle Nutrition, the tenth and last principle. A focus on nutrition in the beginning might have sabotaged your ability to challenge the notion of "good" and "bad" foods. It was important that you learned to view foods as *emotionally equivalent* in order to truly tune in to which foods give you the most satisfaction and feel good in your body. Hopefully, you're now ready to extend that to which foods to include in your world in order to derive the benefit of good health.

Generally, the desire to include nutritious foods in your eating life naturally evolves from achieving competency in the other principles. When people first reject the diet mentality and make peace with food, they often comment that they can't even look at the foods that they were required to eat when dieting. Salads, apples, cottage cheese, broccoli, and grilled skinless chicken breasts are the last things that seem appealing and satisfying to them. But as peace with food is established, along with the clear knowledge that you will never go on another diet, a strange phenomenon emerges. Instead of visions of cotton candy or potato chips or candy bars, people start to truly crave the salad or apple that had been anathema to them only months before!

Why is this? It's the paradox of Intuitive Eating. As a result of full permission, habituation, and sensory specific satiety, the excitement that comes with eating something that is forbidden or restricted vanishes. Foods that you previously ate guiltily and mindlessly never reached that point of habituation, and your taste buds never noticed that the food just didn't taste as good as it did at the start. But once you have full permission, these forbidden foods are no big deal, and they are no longer the golden ring at the merry-go-round that continually calls out to be grabbed. Consequently, the door opens to desiring foods that had been left behind or rebelliously rejected.

In this chapter, you will practice exercises that will

- explain and evaluate your *body-food choice congruence*;

- help you to evaluate your balance of nutritious food and *play food*;

- help you ponder the impact that nutrition might have on your health and on your food choices;

- examine the meaning of *authentic health* and whether you have achieved it;

- explore your food wisdom;

- cultivate an ability to eat sufficient amounts of food for energy and well-being; and

- explore the correlation between nutrition and satisfaction.

Body-Food Choice Congruence

This piece of Intuitive Eating emerges after someone embraces the first nine principles of Intuitive Eating. Body-food choice congruence reflects the principle of gentle nutrition, with an important distinction: it is also a form of interoceptive awareness. It's such an important component that it was added to the updated Intuitive Eating Scale (Tylka and Kroon Van Diest 2013). It represents how foods feel in your body—that is, how eating a particular food or meal makes you feel. This internal awareness causes a shift in how you decide what to eat, going beyond what your taste buds may crave. It means that the tongue is not the only part of the body that we honor when making food choices.

This sets the stage for increased self-care through nutrition, which Gentle Nutrition offers. It is about making food choices based on health and body functioning as well as pleasure. This includes making food choices in order to feel better and to increase energy and body performance. This is not about ignoring the taste buds. Satisfaction is always the engine that leads the Intuitive Eating train. Satisfaction and pleasure in eating can arrive at the station only when you choose foods that tickle your palate and give you joy. It's simply that this isn't the only consideration anymore. How your body feels and works becomes equally important in your food choices, and, in fact, when you feel good, you get even more satisfaction from eating. It doesn't matter how good a food tastes, if you feel lousy after eating it, your entire experience is tainted, and you have diminished satisfaction.

Body-food choice congruence is reflected in many kinds of comments:

- I'd like more energy and stamina.

- I want to get pregnant and want to make sure I'm feeding my baby everything it needs to grow properly and be healthy.

- I sometimes get hungry too soon. I might last longer if I alter my food choice a bit.

- I don't think I'm taking in enough nutritious foods.

- I haven't had a salad for ages, and now I'm really craving one.

- I'd really like to feel better.

Below are questions you can ask when you're ready to find body and food congruence. Do this practice when you're mildly hungry and are thinking about what you would like to eat. As you consider each food option that is appealing to you, work through the following questions.

In the past, how has this food made my body feel while I was eating it?

_____

_____

_____

Did I like this feeling?

_____

_____

How did I feel after I ate?

_____

_____

_____

Would I choose to feel that way again?

_____

_____

Did this food or meal give me lasting, sustainable energy?

_____

_____

The Messages from Your Body

Listen to how you feel physically after eating the foods you choose. Your body will tell you what works for you and what doesn't. Something might look great but make you sleepy or hurt your stomach or cause your blood sugar to drop quickly. It's important to weigh all of these things and not just go simply for the needs of your taste buds.

After you've eaten, consider the following questions:

How did my body feel after eating this food or meal? Did I like this feeling?

_____

_____

Were there any ill effects from my meal—for example, excessive gas or bloating, stomachache, headache, or tiredness? Do I want to repeat this distress?

_____

Did I feel more energy after eating?

_____

Did I feel sufficient satiety from my meal? Did my meal or snack hold me long enough, or did I get hungry too quickly?

_____

In general, are my eating patterns working well for me, or are there some adjustments I need to make?

_____

_____

_____

Remember that Intuitive Eating is a dynamic interplay of instinct, emotion, and thought. If necessary, from time to time, use your rational thinking to help you overcome any glitches in your eating, such as changes in hunger signals or your food choices due to illness or emotions. But also remember to approach this goal with a *for the most part* mentality. Changes in your hunger cues, desires, and other body signals may sometimes happen, and you may choose to act on these changes without overriding them. That's all part of being an Intuitive Eater!

Play Food Versus Nutritious Food

People frequently use the term *junk food* when referring to foods they deem to have inferior value. But when you think about junk, what comes to your mind? Perhaps you think about it meaning something that needs to be thrown in the garbage can or something worthless, without value. As an Intuitive Eater, consider replacing the term *play food* for *junk food*. What comes to mind when thinking about the word *play*? And how does that word make you feel?

_____

_____

Why do kids get weekends off from school? Why do you take vacations or go to the beach on Sunday? If all we ever did were study or work, we would surely burn out. We need rest time, an occasional time-out; we need *playtime* to give us balance in our lives. You can apply the same principle to your eating. If all you ever eat is rigidly healthy food, you risk becoming disordered. There is a recognized disorder called *orthorexia*, the pursuit of and obsession with foods you consider healthy. Doesn't sound very balanced, does it? This is why we propose replacing the term *junk food* with *play food*. Play food is simply food that you crave whose main nutritional value is as an energy source, that is, calories. It usually lacks much in the way of vitamins, minerals, protein, or fiber.

Enjoy yourself—have that cookie or chip. Be assured that having made full peace with food, play food is not all that you'll desire. Plenty of nutritious food will also find its way into your eating world.

Are You Ready to Consider Nutrition in Your Food Choices?

In this section, you will assess your readiness to bring body-food choice congruence into your relationship with food. This will help you know whether your choice for healthy food is coming from a place of true healing and trust or whether you still need to do some more work in making peace with food.

What Motivates Your Food Choice?

The first step in determining your motivation for your food choice is to look at your intention. Are you making your choice for a highly nutritious food based on a true desire for it, to consciously add more nutrients to your food intake, or is it based on a previous food rule? Answer the following questions when you are actually hungry and about to make a food choice. And be sure to answer them spontaneously. Come from your gut when you search for the answer, rather than thinking about what the "right" answer might be.

1. Is the nutritional value of a food the only thing you consider when you find that you're noticing hunger and need to make a decision as to what to eat? _____

   If your answer was yes, reflect upon whether you innately enjoy nutritious food or whether that choice is based on years of being told that you should eat more healthfully. This is not a black-and-white question or answer. You may truly like salads and vegetables and fruits and fish and beans, just as you know that they are all nutritious foods. Just go deeply inside to see if you can find the most authentic answer. In this context, describe your relationship with nutritious food.

   _____

   _____

   _____

   If your answer was that you just go with what your tongue tells you, without regard to the food's nutritional value, reflect on whether you ever think about how the food will feel in your body or what effect it might have on your body after the digestion process begins.

   _____

   _____

   _____

If your answer was that most of the time you choose food based on its nutritional value, but sometimes you choose food just because it will taste good, reflect on your emotional reaction to this philosophy. Does this concept feel like the right fit for you?

_____

_____

_____

2. Examine your emotional relationship with play food. What feelings arise when you choose to eat play food?

_____

_____

_____

_____

_____

_____

How often do you crave play food? Daily? Several times a day? Weekly? Rarely?

_____

How much play food can you eat and still feel well physically? Very little? A medium amount? A lot? (This is subjective—remember to give a gut reaction answer.)

_____

How often do you eat more play food in a sitting or in a day than you know your body can handle—that is, you eat an amount of play food that you know might make you feel queasy, a little sick, bloated, tired, and so forth? Daily? Several times a day? Weekly? Rarely?

_____

_____

Reflect upon your answers to the previous questions to determine your overall approach to the nutritional content of food. Which of the following statements do you agree with (choose as many as apply to you)?

1. You eat nutritious food simply because you think that it's something you should do. Yes _____ No _____

2. You actually enjoy nutritious food because of its taste. Yes _____ No _____

3. You also appreciate its value in your good health. Yes _____ No _____

4. You eat play food when you crave it as long as it doesn't make you feel physically uncomfortable afterward. Yes _____ No _____

5. You eat play food in preference to more nutritious food without regard to its lower nutritional value or how your body reacts to this choice. Yes _____ No _____

If you answered yes to questions 2 through 4, it's likely that your motivation for your food choices comes from a combination of a desire to provide nutritious food for your physical well-being and to have the option of eating something just for its taste. You care about how you feel, as well as wanting to have a satisfying eating experience. You hold no judgment when you choose to eat the foods with the lesser nutritional value, and you're also aware of how your body reacts to the amount of these foods that you eat. You are ready for gentle nutrition!

Authentic Health

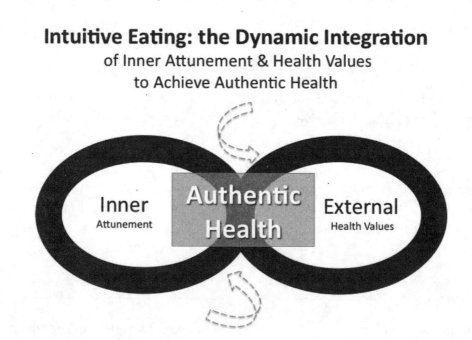

Figure 10.1.   Authentic Health.
Reprinted with permission from Tribole and Resch 2012 / St. Martin's Press.

A healthy eater is one who not only strives for a healthy balance of foods but also has a healthy relationship with food. Your food choices do not elicit a sense of moral superiority or inferiority. In fact, you make no connection between your eating and the essence of who you are as an individual. You simply take a neutral approach to receiving messages from all appropriate sources and integrating them to feel a healthy balance in your life. This process brings you to *authentic health.*

Authentic health is achieved by integrating the messages from your inner world of body and mind with the health guidelines concerning nutrition and movement that come from legitimate sources in the external world, such as the USDA, National Institutes of Health, the FDA, and the US Department of Health and Human Services, among others. Your inner world provides a dynamic interplay of instinct, emotion, and thought. Instinct is ruled by the primitive, survival part of your brain. It provides you with the instinct to eat because you're hungry and to stop because you're full. Unfortunately, instinct can't always help you. Sometimes illness can disconnect you from your hunger signals. Sometimes your emotions can interfere with your hunger and fullness signals. For some people, being anxious or upset blocks their hunger signals. For others, emotions and thoughts can trigger them to eat beyond fullness in order to comfort or numb their emotions. Fortunately, our highest level of brain functioning, which involves the neocortex, is capable of using rational thought to override any potential physical or emotional interference. Working together in this dynamic interplay, your inner world helps you stay attuned to your physical and emotional needs.

Authentic health is achieved by staying attuned to the messages from your body while maintaining sensitivity to external health guidelines prescribed by nutrition experts, based on scientific research and consensus. Your external guidelines can also include philosophical preferences, such as attention to ecology and the environment. You might be concerned with sustainable agriculture, the production of food, fiber, or other plant or animal products using farming techniques that protect the environment, public health, human communities, and animal welfare. You may have a focus on organic food—food produced by farming methods designed to encourage soil and water conservation, reduce pollution, and eliminate the need for artificial pesticides. You may choose to pursue vegetarianism or veganism, whether for their potential health benefits or for personal reasons.

If any of these philosophical or health policy issues speaks to you, it is most important that you are clearly ready to put your attention to the external world while also honoring the messages from your inner world. Any sense that you may be forming a rigid mind-set to any of these new points of views will alert you to the necessity of reevaluating your relationship with food. If that is the case, repeating the exercises dispersed throughout this workbook is the appropriate choice at that time.

You can evaluate whether you are achieving authentic health by answering the following questions:

How do you critically evaluate the source and scientific merit of the nutrition information you receive from the outer world: social media, magazines, friends, family, and so forth? That is, do you look for scientific rationale to support it, do you simply absorb the notions that circulate among your family or friends, or do you just have a gut reaction to what you hear?

_____

_____

_____

_____

If you receive information that seems scientifically valid, do you evaluate how you will feel, physically and emotionally, if you integrate it into your eating life? Might you feel deprived or controlled by it? Will you feel grateful that you've been informed and are willing to make certain sacrifices to change your eating style? Might you feel superior to others who don't eat this way?

_____

_____

_____

_____

If you integrate the information and become anxious as a result, do you reevaluate whether these changes are in your best interest?   Usually _____ Sometimes _____ Never _____

When you hear about the latest nutritional craze, such as avoidance of gluten, GMOs (genetically modified foods), or added sugar, do you consider its potential ill effects to your relationship with food, mind, and body?   Usually _____ Sometimes _____ Never _____

If you reject the craze, do you feel left out when you hear others tout its value?
Usually _____ Sometimes _____ Never _____

When you are feeling stressed out and vulnerable, do you turn to the latest nutrition fad to gain a false sense of power and control over your life?
Usually _____ Sometimes _____ Never _____

Are you able to honor your philosophical preferences (such as considering environmental issues) without becoming rigid about your food choices?
Usually _____ Sometimes _____ Never _____

You have likely achieved authentic health if you

- have evaluated the scientific validity of nutrition guidelines from the external world;

- have integrated some of them into your life without causing anxiety or creating a sense of false control over your life or superiority over others; and

- honor your physical well-being, including staying in touch with your hunger, satiety, and satisfaction.

Food Wisdom

If you are ready to bring more nutrition into your eating life, now is the time to learn and practice the tenets of the food wisdom that Intuitive Eating has to offer you. If reading this information triggers a sense of deprivation, fear, or anxiety, you may not be ready to read this section. You can always come back to it in the future, when you feel more settled into the world of Intuitive Eating.

Starting with the Basics: Variety, Moderation, and Balance

Let's begin with some questions for you to ponder about some basic but very important concepts for healthy eating. (If you begin to roll your eyes, it may be a sign that you're not yet ready to answer these questions.)

When you hear the word *variety*, what comes to your mind? Does it sound like a health care mantra that might be difficult to achieve? Or might the idea of eating a variety of foods make sense to you?

_____

_____

Now think about *moderation*. A boring concept? Or perhaps something that describes the way you eat right now?

_____

_____

_____

How about *balance*? When you hear that word, do you have concerns that each meal needs to be perfectly balanced? Or do you think about balance in broader terms?

_____

_____

Let's begin with *variety*. Generally, we tend to seek variety in our foods so we can get the most enjoyment out of our meals (recall that the pleasantness of a particular food diminishes after a couple of minutes, thanks to sensory specific satiety). Also, the more variety in your daily intake, the more opportunity you have of receiving the abundance of nutrients—protein, fats, carbohydrates, fiber, vitamins, minerals, phytochemicals, and so forth—that foods can offer. If you eat the same food day after day, you limit your exposure to the wide spectrum of these nutrients. Dieting limits the variety of foods and sometimes eliminates entire food groups. There have been eras when low-carb, high-protein diets were popular, followed by periods that favored high carbs and low protein, followed by extremely low fat eras, and on and on.

How can you increase the variety of your foods if you've had a habit of only eating certain allowed foods or if you have become unquestioningly routine in your eating?

_____

_____

_____

_____

_____

In the question of *moderation*, you may have already found that as an Intuitive Eater, you are regularly eating more moderately, because you are honoring hunger and fullness and have made peace with all foods. You have completed the exercises in chapter 7, Cope with Your Feelings Without Using Food, on emotional eating and no longer eat in excess. Some readers, however, might feel that they are not yet consistently eating moderately. On some days, this might be easier, but on other days, they might have problems.

If you're not eating moderately right now, which principles of Intuitive Eating might need some more practice?

_____

_____

Finally, let's look at *balance*. Some people might interpret the concept of eating in a balanced way to mean that each meal must have a complete balance of nutrients. This is not realistic or even necessary. In studies in which toddlers are given free rein to eat a wide variety of foods, without restriction, it is found that over a week's time, they receive everything they need for nutritional health. They end up with enough protein, carbohydrates, fat, vitamins, minerals, and fiber in just the distribution and proportion needed to maintain health (Birch et al. 1991). Adults often become disconnected from their intuitive wisdom due to powerful influences from the media, from friends, and certainly from dieting, but that wisdom can be regained.

Think about a typical week. In that week, do you believe that you get the balance you need? Are there any areas that might need some attention in order to balance out the week?

_____

_____

_____

_____

_____

Nutrition Recommendations

The US Dietary Guidelines are updated and published every five years as a joint effort between the US Department of Health and Human Services and the US Department of Agriculture. (USDHHS and USDA 2015). These guidelines reflect the findings from the current body of nutrition science and are the foundation for nutrition policies and programs throughout the United States. When considering these guidelines, remember that it's important to keep in mind that science evolves, and there are bound to be changes as new research findings emerge. This is why some recommendations seem to conflict with the previous guidelines, which can be confusing to the public—and to nutritionists as well. It's another good reason to strive for variety, moderation, and balance, as that will help you bridge the gaps among the ever-changing recommendations.

In this section, the five overarching 2015–2020 Dietary Guidelines will be highlighted. But as you read them, it's important to remember that your wisdom and gut sense are a vital component. Even the executive summary of the guidelines urges the reader to keep in mind that: "These Guidelines embody the idea that a healthy eating pattern is not a rigid prescription, but rather, an adaptable framework in which individuals can enjoy foods that meet their personal, cultural, and traditional preferences" (USDHHS and USDA 2015, xi). This is a wonderful shift and evolution from previous guidelines.

Before looking at these guidelines, a little nutritional information will explain the basis for some of the recommendations. Our energy intake comes from carbohydrates, protein, and fat. We receive much of our vitamins, minerals, and fiber from fruits, vegetables, whole grains, beans, and nuts.

- Carbohydrates give us our main source of energy, especially for the brain, as carbohydrates are its exclusive energy source. This vital energy source is so important that if you don't get enough of it, your body will cannibalize your muscle by dismantling its protein into amino acids and converting it to glucose (this process is called *gluconeogenesis*, which means "the creation of new sugar").

- Proteins are the building blocks of muscles, organs, hair, nails, enzymes, hormones, and more. Remember, if you don't take in enough carbohydrates, your body will use your protein—both from what you eat and from your own body. This is a very expensive source of energy—both in dollars and in damage to the body!

- Fats are necessary for many functions—for the absorption of our fat-soluble vitamins, for the creation of the myelin sheaths that protects our nerves, for the neurotransmitter receptor sites in our brains, for providing us with satiety and satisfaction in our food, for insulating us to keep us warm and protect our inner organs, and more.

- Vitamins and minerals help to convert food into energy, repair cell damage, strengthen bones, heal wounds, and boost the immune system, and are involved in producing blood cells, hormones, and neurotransmitters associated with mood and cognition, among other functions.

- Fiber helps digestion and is necessary for the healthy functioning of the gastro-intestinal tract.

THE FIVE OVERARCHING 2015–2020 GUIDELINES

Here is a look at the recommendations.

1. *"Follow a healthy eating pattern across the lifespan."* Eating patterns are the combination of foods and drinks that a person eats over time. This speaks to our recommendation for variety. A healthy pattern of eating includes

   - a variety of vegetables, including vegetables of a range of colors, legumes (beans and peas), starchy vegetables, and leafy greens;

   - fruits, especially whole fruits rather than juice;

   - grains, at least half of which are whole grains;

   - dairy, including milk, yogurt, cheese, and fortified soy beverages;

- a variety of protein foods, including seafood, lean meats and poultry, eggs, legumes (beans and peas), soy products, and nuts and seeds; and

- oils, including those from plants and those which are naturally present in nuts, seeds, seafood, olives, and avocados.

2. *"Focus on variety, nutrient density, and amount."* Every food offers its unique set of nutrients. You'll have a better chance of covering all of the bases if you expand your selection of types of foods. *Nutrient density* simply means that you get more bang for your buck by choosing foods that contain more nutrients and energy per ounce. Nutrient-dense foods include nuts and seeds, beans, avocados, salmon, kale, blueberries, and egg yolks, among many others.

3. *"Limit…added sugars…and reduce sodium."* *Added sugars* refers to sugar and corn syrups (as well as most other sweeteners, like honey) that are added to foods in processing or when you prepare foods yourself (such as adding a spoonful of sugar to coffee or tea). It doesn't refer to the naturally occurring sugars in such things as milk and fruits (and some vegetables). (Note—this does not imply that we encourage artificial sweeteners, as they are known to disconnect you from internal satiety and reward cues.) Many highly processed foods, from canned soups to crackers to sandwich meats, are especially high in sodium.

4. *"Shift to healthier food and beverage choices."* This recommendation speaks to choosing foods and drinks that offer more nutritional value. For example, choosing milk or fresh juice over soda; fresh fruits and vegetables over canned vegetables or fruits sitting in syrup; and whole foods over foods that are heavily processed.

5. *"Support healthy eating patterns for all."* The goal of this recommendation is to expand healthy lifestyle choices beyond the home into school, work, and the community through easy, accessible, culturally appropriate, and affordable means.

Eat Not Too Much—and Not Too Little

ISSUES OF EATING NOT TOO MUCH

It is important to note that we have included no portion sizes in this book. Portion size is an issue if you're a distracted, restrictive, or unconscious eater, but it is not a concern for Intuitive Eaters, because they are in touch with fullness and satisfaction. The 2015–2020 Dietary Guidelines stress the "importance of focusing not on individual nutrients or foods in isolation, but on the variety of what people eat and drink—healthy eating patterns as a whole." Yet they do provide calorie targets, which reinforces the dieting mentality and thus is problematic.

ISSUES OF EATING TOO LITTLE

As we discussed earlier, eating enough of a wide variety of foods is necessary for getting the nutrients important for overall health. Many people fall short of this goal. They lack essential vitamins, for instance, because they don't eat enough fresh fruits and vegetables. So below are some suggestions to consider—*for the most part*. These are merely targets to *average* over a period of time. It is *not* a rigid recommendation! And, once again, if looking at these recommendations makes you feel uncomfortable, please skip this section.

Consume enough of these foods:

- Fruits and vegetables—including plenty of dark green leafy vegetables and brightly colored fruits and vegetables, including red and orange varieties.

- Fish—twice a week.

- Carbohydrates—a minimum of 130 grams a day for most adults and teenagers, increased to 175 for women during pregnancy and 210 during lactation. These are emphasized here because they have become widely vilified and feared. Remember, carbohydrates are the exclusive fuel of the brain.

- Nutrient-dense foods.

- Protein-rich foods, including beans, fish, poultry, meat, eggs, dairy, and nuts. Many people get far more protein than they need, but there are some whose protein intake is insufficient.

- Quality fats—omega-3 fats from seafood, fish oil, algae, and seaweed, as well as fats from olive oil, avocado, nuts, seeds, flaxseed oil, and canola oil.

- Whole foods—those which are unprocessed and retain their fiber, vitamins, and minerals.

If you would like more personalized information about your nutritional needs, please contact a registered dietitian nutritionist who is trained in Intuitive Eating. The list of resources at the end of this book contains information on how to locate one.

Take a moment to reflect on the spectrum of foods that you eat in a typical week to see if you are eating an insufficient amount of one or more of these foods. Are there any categories that you have neglected? If so, how might you find a way to bolster your nutrition?

- Do you need to go grocery shopping more often?

- Should you widen the types of restaurants at which you eat?

- Do you need to do a bit more cooking at home?

_____

_____

_____

Above all, remember that Intuitive Eating is the dynamic interplay of instinct, emotion, and thought. If necessary, from time to time, use your rational thinking to help you overcome any glitches you find in your eating—that is, changes in hunger signals or your food choices due to illness, stress or emotions. Also, if you have a medical condition, be sure to consult with a registered dietitian or nutritionist trained in Intuitive Eating for medical nutrition therapy. Making decisions about how to eat based on true medical needs and Intuitive Eating are not mutually exclusive.

For your day-to-day decisions about how to eat, always remember that you were born with the instinct to eat what you need to nourish your body. Intuitive Eating is about guiding you back to that place, stripping you of restrictive thinking and emotional eating. Be assured that you can take in nutrition guidelines without them becoming a new set of rules and restrictions; you can use the information they contain while knowing that your body will inform you of what you truly need to get variety, moderation, and balance in your eating.

Nutrition and Satisfaction

In chapter 6, Discover the Satisfaction Factor, you practiced many exercises to help you find the foods that are most satisfying to you. At this point, we're adding one more consideration in your quest for eating satisfaction—nutrition. Be aware that for some people, this discussion on nutrition triggers old feelings about the foods they _should_ choose or restrict—these thoughts are evidence of a lingering diet mentality. Take a moment to check in with yourself to see if this has happened and to immediately challenge those thoughts:

_____

_____

_____

Remember that satisfaction is the driving force in Intuitive Eating. If you keep the goal of satisfaction regularly in your mind, you will be motivated not only to honor all the Intuitive Eating principles but also to find a way to include sufficient nutritious food in your weekly food choices to honor your health. If you feel more satisfied in your meal by including some highly nutritious food, by all means, include it. Maintaining a balance of nutritious food with some play food may be the best path to a lifetime of satisfying eating. Just be sure that you listen to the messages that your body gives you about your food choices and that you hold no judgment when you choose to eat the foods with lesser nutritional value.

Wrap-Up

It Doesn't Have to Be Perfect

Sometimes you won't have the option to get just what you want. Maybe you choose to eat at a friend's or relative's house for the joy of socializing, but this person is not a very good cook. Or you might travel to a country whose cuisine is not appealing to you or which doesn't have the availability of the fresh and nutritious foods your prefer. Or you might unexpectedly find yourself stuck without the food you enjoy eating and have to make do with what's available. It's important to remember that there are many meals ahead of you—in fact, there's one about every three or four hours. You will have many more opportunities for finding satisfaction and the types of foods that fit your nutritional preferences. No one meal—or even weeks of meals, if you're on an extended trip—will affect your overall nutrition. Intuitive Eating is not about perfection—it's simply about offering you guidelines for a comfortable relationship with food.

So, relax. Remember that the concept *for the most part* is central. For the most part, strive for variety, moderation, and balance in your eating. For the most part, enjoy both nutritious foods and some play foods. For the most part, eat satisfying meals. The calm and trust that you feel about food, based on your inner wisdom and refusal to strive for perfection, will carry you through a lifetime of freedom and joy in your eating!

You have now practiced many exercises connected to all ten principles of Intuitive Eating. As a result, we hope that you have found a deeper understanding of what Intuitive Eating means and a deep trust that if you listen carefully to all of the messages your body and inner wisdom provide for you, you will know just what to eat, when to eat, and how much to eat. You may need to go back to some of the exercises in this workbook in order to hone your Intuitive Eating skills. The more you practice, the closer you will find yourself to a world free from dieting and full of pleasurable eating, self-respect, and self-esteem!

Intuitive Eating Resources

General

Intuitive Eating Book

Tribole, E., and E. Resch, 2012. *Intuitive Eating*, 3rd edition. St. Martin's Press: NY, NY.

Intuitive Eating Audio CD

This set of four CDs, which is an excellent companion to our book, focuses on the practical how-to aspects of Intuitive Eating. It is not a verbatim reading of the book.

Intuitive Eating Website

http://www.intuitiveeating.org

Get the latest news from our blog and calendar of events. You will also find articles, research, interviews, and general information about Intuitive Eating.

Counseling and Support

Certified Intuitive Eating Counselor Directory

http://www.intuitiveeatingcounselordirectory.org

This is a listing of allied health professionals who are trained and certified in the Intuitive Eating process. We receive numerous requests for local Intuitive Eating health professionals. To help fill this gap, we offer certification for allied health professionals. These health professionals include dietitians, psychotherapists, physicians, physical therapists, nurses, chiropractors, dentists, occupational therapists, licensed massage therapists, licensed physical trainers, certified health education specialists, licensed health and life coaches, and others in the health profession who espouse the Intuitive Eating principles in their work.

Intuitive Eating Online Community

http://www.intuitiveeatingcommunity.org

Be inspired, share your story, and partake of the many tools to empower your Intuitive Eating journey. This is your community, with over ten thousand members. It's free, but you will need to sign up.

Professional Resources

How to Become a Certified Intuitive Eating Counselor

We are eager to spread the message of Intuitive Eating through allied health professionals who qualify to be certified and listed on our Intuitive Eating Counselor Directory. Training for this certification includes three steps:

1. A self-study program administered by Helm Publishing (http://www.helmpublishing.com).

2. Intuitive Eating PRO teleseminar training, led by Evelyn Tribole.

3. Supervision and coaching with either Elyse Resch or Evelyn Tribole.

Upon completion of the certification requirements, you will have the option to receive the following:

1. Membership in the Certified Intuitive Eating Counselors Community.

2. Listing in the Certified Intuitive Eating Counselors Directory on the Intuitive Eating website (http://www.intuitiveeating.org).

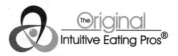

Figure R.1.   The logo of certified Intuitive Eating counselors.

For more details and information see these websites:

http://www.evelyntribole.com

http://www.elyseresch.com

http://www.intuitiveeatingprotraining.com

http://www.helmpublishing.com

Intuitive Eating Professionals on LinkedIn

http://bit.ly/LinkedIn-IEPro

An international group of nearly four thousand allied health professionals. We share news, views, and resources.

References

Adams, C., and M. Leary. 2007. "Promoting Self-Compassionate Attitudes Toward Eating Among Restrictive and Guilty Eaters." *Journal of Social and Clinical Psychology* 26 (10): 1120–44.

Albertson, E., K. Neff, and K. Dill-Shackleford. 2015. "Self-Compassion and Body Dissatisfaction in Women: A Randomized Controlled Trial of a Brief Meditation Intervention." *Mindfulness.* 6 (3): 444–54.

Avalos, L., T. Tylka, and N. Wood-Barcalow. 2005. "The Body Appreciation Scale: Development and Psychometric Evaluation." *Journal of Body Image* 2: 285–297.

Bacon, L., and L. Aphramor. 2011. "Weight Science: Evaluating the Evidence for a Paradigm Shift." *Nutrition Journal* 10: 9. DOI: 10.1186/1475–2891–10–9.

Barnes, R., and S. Tantleff-Dunn. 2010. "Food for Thought: Examining the Relationship Between Food Thought Suppression and Weight-Related Outcomes." *Eating Behaviors* 11 (3): 175–79.

Barnett, J., K. Baker, N. Elman, and G. Schoener. 2007. "In Pursuit of Wellness: The Self-Care Imperative." *Professional Psychology: Research and Practice* 38 (6): 603–12.

Birch, L. L. and M. Deysher. 1986. "Calorie Compensation and Sensory Specific Satiety: Evidence for Self-Regulation of Food Intake by Young Children." *Appetite* 7 (4): 323–31.

Birch, L. L., S. L. Johnson, G, Andresen, J. C. Peters, M. C. Schulte. 1991. "The Variability of Young Children's Energy Intake." *New England Journal of Medicine* 324 (4): 232–23. DOI: 10.1056/NEJM199101243240405.

Brunstrom, J., and G. Mitchell. 2006. "Effects of Distraction on the Development of Satiety." *British Journal of Nutrition.* 96 (4): 761–69.

Calogero, R., and K. Pedrotty. 2007. "Daily Practices for Mindful Exercise." In *Handbook of Low-Cost Preventive Interventions for Physical and Mental Health: Theory, Research, and Practice*, edited by L. L'Abate, D. Embry, and M. Baggett, 141–60. New York: Springer-Verlag.

Cameron, J., G. Goldfield, G. Finlayson, J. Blundell, and E. Doucet. 2014. "Fasting for 24 Hours Heightens Reward from Food and Food-Related Cues." *PLoS ONE* 9 (1): e85970. DOI: 10.1371/journal.pone.0085970.

Carr, K. 2011. "Food Scarcity, Neuroadaptations, and the Pathogenic Potential of Dieting in an Unnatural Ecology: Binge Eating and Drug Abuse." *Physiology and Behavior* 104: 162–67.

Cheval, B., P. Sarrazin, and L. Pelletier. 2014. "Impulsive Approach Tendencies Towards Physical Activity and Sedentary Behaviors, but Not Reflective Intentions, Prospectively Predict Non-Exercise Activity Thermogenesis." *PLoS ONE* 9 (12): e115238. DOI: 10.1371/journal. pone.0115238.

Cook-Cottone, C. 2015. *Mindfulness and Yoga for Self-Regulation: A Primer for Mental Health Professionals.* New York: Springer Publishing Company.

Cook-Cottone, C., E. Tribole, and T. Tylka. 2013. *Healthy Eating in Schools.* Washington, D.C.: American Psychological Association.

Cornil, Y. and P. Chandon. 2015. "Pleasure as an Ally of Healthy Eating? Contrasting Visceral and Epicurean Eating Pleasure and Their Association with Portion Size Preferences and Well-Being." *Appetite* 104: 52–9. DOI: 10.1016/j.appet.2015.08.045.

Craft, L., T. Zderic, S. Gapstur, E. VanIterson, D. Thomas, J. Siddique, and M. Hamilton. 2012. "Evidence That Women Meeting Physical Activity Guidelines Do Not Sit Less: An Observational Inclinometry Study." *The International Journal of Behavioral Nutrition and Physical Activity* 9: 122. http://doi.org/10.1186/1479–5868–9-122.

De Witt Huberts, J., C. Evers, and D. de Ridder. 2013. "Double Trouble: Restrained Eaters Do Not Eat Less and Feel Worse." *Psychology and Health* 28 (6): 686–700.

Dulloo, A., J. Jacquet, and J. Montani. 2012. "How Dieting Makes Some Fatter: From a Perspective of Human Body Composition Autoregulation." *Proceedings of the Nutrition Society* 71: 379–89.

Ekkekakis, P., G. Parfitt, and S. Petruzzello. 2012. "The Pleasure and Displeasure People Feel When They Exercise at Different Intensities Decennial Update and Progress Towards a Tripartite Rationale for Exercise Intensity Prescription." *Sports Medicine* 41 (8): 641–71.

Emmons, R., and E. McCullough. 2003. "Counting Blessings Versus Burdens: An Experimental Investigation of Gratitude and Subjective Well-Being in Daily Life." *Journal of Personality and Social Psychology.* 84 (2): 377–89.

Epstein, L., J. Temple, J. Roemmich, and M. Bouton. 2009. "Habituation as a Determinant of Human Food Intake." *Psychological Review* 116 (2): 384–407. DOI: 10.1037/a0015074.

Field, A., S. Austin, C. Taylor, S. Malspeis, B. Rosner, H. Rockett, and G. Colditz. 2003. "Relation Between Dieting and Weight Change Among Preadolescents and Adolescents." *Pediatrics* 112: 900–906.

Fothergill, E., J. Guo, L. Howard, J. Kerns, N. Knuth, R.Brychta, K. Chen, M. Skarulis, M. Walter, P. Walter, and K. Hall. 2016. "Persistent Metabolic Adaptation 6 Years After 'The Biggest Loser' Competition." *Obesity Biology and Integrated Physiology* 24 (8): 1612–9. http://dx.doi.org/10.1002/oby.21538.

Friedemann Smith C., C. Heneghan, and A. Ward. 2015. "Moving Focus from Weight to Health. What Are the Components Used in Interventions to Improve Cardiovascular Health in Children?" *PLOS One* 10 (8): e0135115. http://dx.doi.org/10.1371/journal.pone.0135115.

Galloway A., C. Farrow, and D. Martz. 2010. "Retrospective Reports of Child Feeding Practices, Current Eating Behaviors and BMI in College Students." *Obesity* 18: 1330–35.

Gearhardt, A., W. Corbin, and K. Brownell. 2009. "Preliminary Validation of the Yale Food Addiction Scale." *Appetite* 52: 430–36.

Grecucci, A., E. Pappaianni, R. Siugzdaite, A. Theuninck, and R. Job. 2015. "Mindful Emotion Regulation: Exploring the Neurocognitive Mechanisms Behind Mindfulness." *BioMed Research International* 670724. http://doi.org/10.1155/2015/670724.

Hainer, V., and I. Aldhoon-Hainerova. 2013. "Obesity Paradox Does Exist." *Diabetes Care* 36(Suppl 2): S276–S281.

Hallowell, E. 2007. *CrazyBusy: Overstretched, Overbooked, and About to Snap! Strategies for Handling Your Fast-Paced Life.* New York, NY: Ballantine Books.

Hamilton, M., D. Hamilton, and T. Zderic. 2004. "Exercise Physiology Versus Inactivity Physiology: An Essential Concept for Understanding Lipoprotein Lipase Regulation." *Exercise and Sport Sciences Reviews* 32 (4): 161–66.

Harned, M., L. Dimeff, E. Woodcock, T. Kelly, J. Zavertnik , I. Contreras, and S. Danner. 2014. "Exposing Clinicians to Exposure: A Randomized Controlled Dissemination Trial of Exposure Therapy for Anxiety Disorders." *Behavior Therapy* 45 (6): 731–44.

Harrington, M., S. Gibson, and R. Cottrell. 2009. "A Review and Meta-Analysis of the Effect of Weight Loss on All-Cause Mortality Risk." *Nutrition Research Reviews* 22 (01): 93–108.

Hetherington, M., B. J. Rolls, and J. Burley. 1989. "The Time Course of Sensory-Specific Satiety." *Appetite* 12 (1): 57–68.

Henson, J., D. Dunstan, M. Davies, and T. Yates. 2016. "Sedentary Behaviour As a New Behavioural Target in the Prevention and Treatment of Type 2 Diabetes." *Diabetes/Metabolism Research and Reviews* 32 (Suppl. 1): 213–20.

Herbert, B., J. Blechert, M. Hautzinger, E. Matthias, and C. Herbert. 2013. "Intuitive Eating Is Associated with Interoceptive Sensitivity. Effects on Body Mass Index." *Appetite* 70:22–30.

Herbert, B., E. Muth, O. Pollatos, and C. Herbert. 2012. "Interoception Across Modalities: On the Relationship Between Cardiac Awareness and the Sensitivity for Gastric Functions." *PLOS One* 7 (5): e36646.

Herman, C., and J. Polivy. 1984. "A Boundary Model for the Regulation of Eating." In *Eating and Its Disorders*, edited by A. Stunkard and E. Stellar, 151. New York, NY: Raven Press.

Holmes, M., M. Fuller-Tyszkiewicz, H. Skouteris, and J. Broadbent. 2014. "Improving Prediction of Binge Episodes by Modelling Chronicity of Dietary Restriction." *European Eating Disorders Review* 22: 405–11.

Ihuoma, U. E., P. A. Crum, and T. L. Tylka. 2008. "The Trust Model: A Different Feeding Paradigm for Managing Childhood Obesity." *Obesity* 16 (10) 2197–204. DOI: 10.1038/oby.2008.378.

Jansen, E., S. Mulkens, and A. Jansen. 2007. "Do Not Eat the Red Food! Prohibition of Snacks Leads to Their Relatively Higher Consumption in Children." *Appetite* 49: 572–77.

Jansen, E., S. Mulkens, A. Emond, and A. Jansen. 2008. "From the Garden of Eden to the Land of Plenty. Restriction of Fruit and Sweets Intake Leads to Increased Fruit and Sweets Consumption in Children." *Appetite* 51 (3): 570–75.

Keeler, C., R. Mattes, and S. Tan. 2015. "Anticipatory and Reactive Responses to Chocolate Restriction in Frequent Chocolate Consumers." *Obesity* 23 (6): 1130–35.

Køster-Rasmussen, R., M. Simonsen, V. Siersma, J. Henriksen, B. Heitmann, and N. Olivarius. 2016. "Intentional Weight Loss and Longevity in Overweight Patients with Type 2 Diabetes: A Population-Based Cohort Study." *PLOS One* 11 (1): e0146889. http://dx.doi.org/10.1371/journal.pone.014688.

Kristeller, J., and R. Wolever. 2011. "Mindfulness-Based Eating Awareness Training for Treating Binge Eating Disorder: The Conceptual Foundation." *Eating Disorders* 19 (1): 49–61.

Lavie, C. 2014. *The Obesity Paradox: When Thinner Means Sicker and Heavier Means Healthier.* New York: Hudson Street Press.

Levine, J., M. Vander Weg, J. Hill, and R. Klesges. 2006. "Non-Exercise Activity Thermogenesis: The Crouching Tiger Hidden Dragon of Societal Weight Gain." *Arteriosclerosis, Thrombosis, and Vascular Biology* 26: 729–36.

Long, C., J. Blundell, and G. Finlayson. 2015. "A Systematic Review of the Application and Correlates of YFAS-Diagnosed 'Food Addiction' in Humans: Are Eating-Related 'Addictions' a Cause for Concern or Empty Concepts?" *European Journal of Obesity* 3: 386–401.

Mann, T. 2015. *Secrets From the Eating Lab.* New York: Harper Collins.

Massey, A. and A. Hill. 2012. "Dieting and Food Craving. A Descriptive, Quasi-Prospective Study." *Appetite* 58 (3): 781–85.

Neal, D., W. Wood, M. Wu, and D. Kurlander. 2011. "The Pull of the Past: When Do Habits Persist Despite Conflict with Motives?" *Personality and Social Psychology Bulletin* 37 (11): 1428–37.

Neff, K. 2003. "Self-Compassion: An Alternative Conceptualization of a Healthy Attitude Toward Oneself." *Self and Identity* 2: 85–101.

———. 2016. "The Self-Compassion Scale Is a Valid and Theoretically Coherent Measure of Self-Compassion." *Mindfulness* 7 (1): 264–74.

Neff, K., and A. Costigan. 2014. "Self-Compassion, Well-being, and Happiness." *Psychologie in Österreich* 2/3: 114–19.

Neumark-Sztainer, D., M. Wall, N. Arson, M. Eisenberg, and K. Loth. 2011. "Dieting and Disordered Eating Behaviors from Adolescence to Young Adulthood: Findings from a 10-Year Longitudinal Study." *Journal of the American Dietetic Association* 111: 1004–11.

Ozier, A., O. Kendrick, L. Knol, J. Leeper, M. Perko, and J. Burnham. 2007. "The Eating and Appraisal Due to Emotions and Stress (EADES) Questionnaire: Development and Validation." *Journal of the American Dietetic Association* 107 (4): 619–28.

Paddock, N. 2014. "Alcohol Disrupts Body's Sleep Regulator." *Medical News Today*. December 11.

Parfitt G., H. Evans, and R. Eston 2012. "Perceptually Regulated Training at RPE13 Is Pleasant and Improves Physical Health." *Medicine and Science in Sports and Exercise* 44 (8): 1613–18. DOI: 10.1249/MSS.0b013e31824d266e.

Péneau S., E. Ménard, C. Méjean, F. Bellisle, S. Hercberg. 2003. "Sex and Dieting Modify the Association Between Emotional Eating and Weight Status." *American Journal of Clinical Nutrition* 97: 1307–13.

Petruzzello, S. 2012. "Doing What Feels Good (and Avoiding What Feels Bad)—A Growing Recognition of the Influence of Affect on Exercise Behavior: A Comment on Williams et al." *Annals of Behavior Medicine* 44 (1): 7–9.

Pietilainen, K., S. Saarni, J. Kaprio, and A. Rissanen. 2012. "Does Dieting Make You Fat? A Twin Study." *International Journal of Obesity* 36: 456–64.

Rezende, L., T. Sa, G. Mielke, J. Viscondi, J. Rey-Lopez, and L. Garcia. 2016. "All-Cause Mortality Attributable to Sitting Time." *American Journal of Preventive Medicine* 51 (2): 253–63.

Robinson, E., P. Aveyard, A. Daley, K. Jolly, A. Lewis, D. Lycett, and S. Higgs. 2013. "Eating Attentively: A Systematic Review and Meta-Analysis of the Effect of Food Intake Memory and Awareness on Eating." *American Journal of Clinical Nutrition* 97: 728–42.

Rolls, B. J. 1986. "Sensory-Specific Satiety." *Nutrition Reviews* 44 (3): 93–101. DOI: 10.1111/j.1753–4887.1986.tb07593.x.

Ross, R., S. Blair, L. de Lannoy, J. Després, and C. Lavie. 2015. "Changing the Endpoints for Determining Effective Obesity Management." *Progress in Cardiovascular Disease* 57 (4): 330–36.

Schoenefeld, S., and J. Webb. 2013. Self-Compassion and Intuitive Eating in College Women: Examining the Contributions of Distress Tolerance and Body Image Acceptance and Action. *Eating Behaviors* 14: 493–96.

Segar, M., J. Eccles, and C. Richardson. 2011. "Rebranding Exercise: Closing the Gap Between Values and Behavior." *International Journal of Behavioral Nutrition and Physical Activity* 8: 94. https://ijbnpa.biomedcentral.com/articles/10.1186/1479–5868-8-94.

Stice, E., K. Burger, and S. Yokum. 2013. "Caloric Deprivation Increases Responsivity of Attention and Reward Brain Regions to Intake, Anticipated Intake, and Images of Palatable Food." *NeuroImage* 67: 322–30.

Stice, E., K. Davis, N. Miller, and C. Marti. 2008. "Fasting Increases Risk for Onset of Binge Eating and Bulimic Pathology: A 5-Year Prospective Study." *Journal of Abnormal Psychology* 117 (4): 941–46.

Tomiyama, A., J. Hunger, J. Nguyen-Cuu, and C. Wells. 2016. "Misclassification of Cardiometabolic Health When Using Body Mass Index Categories in NHANES 2005–2012." *International Journal of Obesity* 40: 883–86. DOI: 10.1038/ijo.2016.17 .

Tomiyama, A., T. Mann, D. Vinas, J. Hunger, J. Dejager, and S. Taylor. 2010. "Low Calorie Dieting Increases Cortisol." *Psychosomatic Medicine* 72 (4): 357–64.

Tribole, E., and E. Resch. 1995. *Intuitive Eating.* 1st ed. New York: St. Martin's Press.

———. 2012. *Intuitive Eating.* 3rd ed. New York: St. Martin's Press.

Truong, G., D. Turk, and T. Handy. 2013. "An Unforgettable Apple: Memory and Attention for Forbidden Objects." *Cognitive, Affective, and Behavioral Neuroscience* 13 (4): 803–13.

Tsafou, K., D. De Ridder, R. van Ee, J. Lacroix. 2015. "Mindfulness and Satisfaction in Physical Activity: A Cross-Sectional Study in the Dutch Population." *Journal of Health Psychology.* DOI: 10.1177/1359105314567207.

Tylka, T. 2006. "Development and Psychometric Evaluation of a Measure of Intuitive Eating." *Journal of Counseling Psychology* 53: 226–40.

Tylka, T., and A. Kroon Van Diest. 2013. "The Intuitive Eating Scale–2: Item Refinement and Psychometric Evaluation with College Women and Men." *Journal of Counseling Psychology* 60 (1): 137–53.

Tylka, T., R. Annunziato, D. Burgard, S. Daníelsdóttir, E. Shuman, C. Davis, and R. Calogero. 2014. "The Weight-Inclusive Versus Weight-Normative Approach to Health: Evaluating the Evidence for Prioritizing Well-Being over Weight Loss." *Journal of Obesity,* article ID 983495, http://dx.doi.org/10.1155/2014/983495.

Tylka, T. and N. L. Wood-Barcalow. 2015. "The Body Appreciation Scale–2: Item Refinement and Psychometric Evaluation." *Body Image.* 12: 53–67.

Urbszat, D., C. Herman, and J. Polivy. 2002. "Eat, Drink, and Be Merry, For Tomorrow We Diet: Effects of Anticipated Deprivation on Food Intake in Restrained and Unrestrained Eaters." *Journal of Abnormal Psychology* 111 (2): 396–401.

USDHHS 2008. *Physical Activity Guidelines.* www.health.gov/paguidelines.

USDHHS and USDA. 2015. *Dietary Guidelines for Americans 2015–2020.* 8th ed. Available at http://health.gov/dietaryguidelines/2015/guidelines.

Wegner, D., D. Schneider, S. Carter, and T. White. 1987. "Paradoxical Effects of Thought Suppression." *Journal of Personality and Social Psychology* 53 (1): 5–13.

Wenzlaff, R., and D. Wegner. 2000. "Thought Suppression." *Annual Review of Psychology* 51: 59–91.

World Health Organization. 2006. Constitution of the World Health Organization—Basic Documents, 45th ed., Supplement, October.

World Health Organization. 2010. *Global Recommendations on Physical Activity for Health.* Geneva, Switzerland: WHO Press.

Wood A., J. Maltby, R. Gillett, P. Linley, and S. Joseph. 2008. "The Role of Gratitude in the Development of Social Support, Stress, and Depression: Two Longitudinal Studies." *Journal of Research in Personality* 42 (4): 854–71.

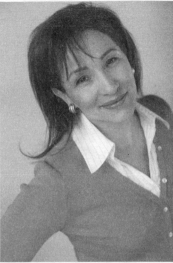

Mikel Healey Photography

Evelyn Tribole, MS, RDN, is an award-winning registered dietitian with a nutrition counseling practice in Newport Beach, CA, specializing in eating disorders. She also trains health professionals on how to help their clients cultivate a healthy relationship with food, mind, and body through the process of Intuitive Eating, a concept she co-pioneered. Tribole is author of several books, including *Healthy Homestyle Cooking*, and is coauthor of *Intuitive Eating*. She was the nutrition expert for *Good Morning America*, and was a national spokesperson for the Academy of Nutrition and Dietetics for six years. She served three years on the Social Media committee of the Academy for Eating Disorders. Tribole is often sought after by the media for her nutritional expertise, and has appeared in hundreds of interviews, including CNN, NBC's *Today Show*, MSNBC, Fox News, *USA Today*, *The Wall Street Journal*, and *People* magazine. She also gives presentations around the world on intuitive eating.

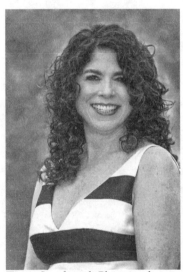

Tracey Landworth Photography

Elyse Resch, MS, RDN, is a nutrition therapist in private practice in Beverly Hills, CA, with over thirty-five years of experience, specializing in eating disorders, intuitive eating, and health at every size. She is coauthor of *Intuitive Eating*, has published journal articles, and does regular speaking engagements and extensive media interviews. Her work has been profiled on CNN, KABC, NBC, AP Press KFI Radio, *USA Today*, and KTTV television, among others. Resch is nationally known for her work in helping patients break free from the diet mentality through the intuitive eating process. Her philosophy embraces the goal of reconnecting with your internal wisdom about eating. She supervises and trains health professionals, is a certified eating disorder registered dietitian, fellow of the International Association of Eating Disorder Professionals, and fellow of the Academy of Nutrition and Dietetics.

Foreword writer **Tracy Tylka, PhD,** is professor of psychology at the Columbus and Marion campuses of The Ohio State University. She attended the University of Akron for her undergraduate and graduate studies, earning her BA in psychology in 1995, MA in counseling psychology in 1998, and PhD in counseling psychology in 2001. Tylka completed her predoctoral internship at the counseling center at Southern Illinois University at Carbondale. She joined the department of psychology at The Ohio State University as an assistant professor in 2001, received tenure and promotion to associate professor in 2007, and was promoted to full professor in 2013.

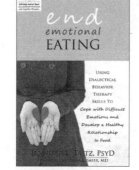
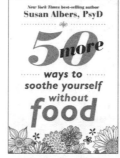
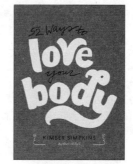
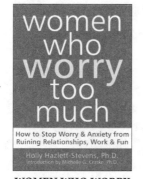
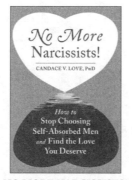
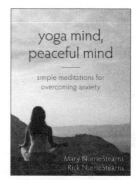
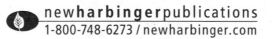

Register your **new harbinger** titles for additional benefits!

When you register your **new harbinger** title—purchased in any format, from any source—you get access to benefits like the following:

- Downloadable accessories like printable worksheets and extra content

- Instructional videos and audio files

- Information about updates, corrections, and new editions

Not every title has accessories, but we're adding new material all the time.

Access free accessories in 3 easy steps:

1. Sign in at NewHarbinger.com (or **register** to create an account).

2. Click on **register a book**. Search for your title and click the **register** button when it appears.

3. Click on the **book cover or title** to go to its details page. Click on **accessories** to view and access files.

That's all there is to it!

If you need help, visit:

NewHarbinger.com/accessories

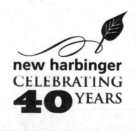

new harbinger
CELEBRATING
40 YEARS